Sweet Spot for Brain Health

Why Blood Sugar Matters for a Clear, Fog-Free Brain

Dr Sui H. Wong MD FRCP

EBH Press. EBHpress.com

Copyright © Dr Sui H. Wong, 2024

ISBN: 978-1-917353-83-0 (E-book), 978-1-917353-84-7 (Paperback), 978-1-917353-85-4 (Hardcover) 978-1-917353-86-1 (Audiobook)

Table of Contents

INTRODUCTION 1

OBJECTIVES OF THIS BOOK 1
THE RELEVANCE OF BLOOD GLUCOSE AND BRAIN HEALTH 2

THEME 1: 5

HOW DOES IT WORK? 5

CHAPTER 1: UNDERSTANDING THE BRAIN-GLUCOSE CONNECTION 7

THE BASICS OF BRAIN METABOLISM 7
    Glucose as the Primary Fuel 7
    Brain Energy Consumption 8
BRAIN FUNCTION AND GLUCOSE DEPENDENCY 8
    Cognitive Performance and Glucose Levels 8
YOUR BODY'S BLOOD SUGAR BALANCING ACT 9
    Glucose Sensing in the Brain 10
BLOOD-BRAIN BARRIER INTEGRITY AND GLUCOSE LEVELS 11
KEY TAKEAWAYS 12

CHAPTER 2: INTO THE BRAIN CELLS 13

NEUROBIOLOGY OF GLUCOSE METABOLISM 13
    Glucose Metabolism Pathways 14
BRAIN ENERGY DEMANDS 16
    Resting vs. Active Brain Glucose Needs 16
    Cognitive Demands and Glucose Metabolism 17
GLUCOSE, OXIDATIVE STRESS, AND BRAIN HEALTH 17
    Mitochondrial Antioxidant Defense 18
    Antioxidant Defense Mechanisms in the Brain 19
KETONES VS. GLUCOSE: ALTERNATIVE BRAIN FUELS 19
    Comparison of Ketones and Glucose 20
KEY TAKEAWAYS 21

CHAPTER 3: IDENTIFYING BLOOD GLUCOSE IMBALANCES 23

UNDERSTANDING GLYCEMIC VARIABILITY 23
    Factors Influencing Glycemic Variability 24
    Glycemic Variability and Health Outcomes 24
HYPOGLYCEMIA: CAUSES AND SYMPTOMS 25
    Symptoms and Immediate Management 26
HYPERGLYCEMIA: RECOGNIZING THE WARNING SIGNS 27
    Hyperglycemia in Non-Diabetics 27
METABOLIC HEALTH 28
    Navigating Insulin Resistance and Metabolic Health 28
BLOOD GLUCOSE TESTING METHODS 30
KEY TAKEAWAYS 31

CHAPTER 4: MENTAL HEALTH, MOOD, AND BLOOD GLUCOSE 33

BLOOD GLUCOSE AND EMOTIONAL REGULATION 33
    Nurturing Emotional Resilience through Balanced Blood Glucose 34
BLOOD SUGAR BALANCE AND STRESS RESPONSE 34
DIETARY SUGARS AND DEPRESSION 36
    Sugar Consumption and Inflammation 37
    Impact on Gut Microbiome 38
KEY TAKEAWAYS 39

THEME 2: 41

WHEN THINGS GO WRONG 41

CHAPTER 5: THE LONG-TERM EFFECTS OF DYSREGULATED BLOOD GLUCOSE ON
BRAIN HEALTH 43

CHRONIC HYPERGLYCEMIA AND COGNITIVE DECLINE 43
INSULIN RESISTANCE AND ITS IMPACT ON THE BRAIN 44
    Insulin Resistance and Alzheimer's Disease 44
VASCULAR HEALTH, BLOOD GLUCOSE, AND THE BRAIN 45
    Impact of Glycemic Variability on Cerebral Blood Flow 46
    Preventive Strategies for Vascular Health 47
PREVENTING BRAIN ATROPHY WITH BLOOD GLUCOSE CONTROL 48
IMPACT OF BLOOD GLUCOSE ON MITOCHONDRIAL HEALTH IN THE BRAIN 49
    Therapeutic Approaches Targeting Mitochondria 50
KEY TAKEAWAYS 51

THEME 3: **53**

PRACTICAL STRATEGIES FOR BLOOD SUGAR REGULATION TO ENHANCE BRAIN HEALTH **53**

CHAPTER 6: DIET AND ITS IMPACT ON BRAIN ENERGY **55**

UNDERSTANDING THE GLYCEMIC INDEX 55

Low-GI Foods 56

Medium-GI Foods 56

High-GI Foods 56

Glycemic Load and Brain Function 57

BALANCING MACRONUTRIENTS FOR OPTIMAL BRAIN ENERGY 58

Carbohydrates for Sustained Energy 58

Fiber 59

Healthy Fats and Cognitive Health 59

Proteins for the Brain and Satiety 61

Personalizing Your Healthy Eating Plate 62

MORE NUTRITION TIPS FOR STABILIZING YOUR BLOOD SUGAR 63

Impact of Meal Patterns on Brain Energy 63

Mindful Snacking 64

Choose Vegetables First 64

Save Desserts for Last 64

Portion Sizes 65

Make Resistant Starch 65

Reduce your AGE 65

Flaxseed and Blueberries 66

Vinegar 66

Limit Ultra-Processed Foods 66

Pre-Plan your Shopping Trip 67

ADDITIONAL CONSIDERATIONS 67

Ketogenic Diet and Brain Metabolism 67

Hydration for Your Brain and Blood Sugar 68

High-Mercury Fish 70

Glucose Checks and Medication Review 70

KEY TAKEAWAYS 71

CHAPTER 7: LIFESTYLE CHOICES FOR OPTIMAL BRAIN FUNCTION **73**

EXERCISE AND PHYSICAL ACTIVITY FOR BRAIN AND GLUCOSE BENEFITS 73

Types of Exercise and Their Effects on Brain and Blood Glucose 74

Impact of Exercise and Physical Activity on Brain Health and Neurogenesis 75

Incorporating Exercise and Physical Activity into a Regular Routine 76

SLEEP'S ROLE IN GLUCOSE REGULATION AND BRAIN HEALTH 78

Sleep Deprivation and Glucose Metabolism 78

Circadian Rhythms and Glucose Control 79

Sleep Quality and Cognitive Recovery 79

Impact of Sleep on Willpower and Decision-Making 80

Strategies for Improving Sleep Quality 80

Recognizing and Addressing Sleep Disorders 81

MINDFULNESS AND COGNITIVE FUNCTION 83

Mindfulness in Managing Cravings and Making Healthier Choices 84

THE IMPACT OF ALCOHOL AND CAFFEINE ON BRAIN GLUCOSE LEVELS 85

Alcohol, Hypoglycemia, and Brain Health 85

Caffeine, Glucose Metabolism, and Cognitive Alertness 85

Nicotine's Effect on Insulin and Glucose Control 86

Moderation and Balance in Consumption 86

KEY TAKEAWAYS 87

CHAPTER 8: NATURAL REMEDIES AND SUPPLEMENTS 91

ANTIOXIDANTS AND BRAIN PROTECTION 91

HERBS AND SPICES FOR BLOOD GLUCOSE CONTROL 92

Cinnamon 92

Ginseng 93

Berberine 94

Moringa 94

OMEGA-3 FATTY ACIDS AND BRAIN FUNCTION 94

Marine Sources 95

Plant-Based Sources 95

PROBIOTICS, GUT HEALTH, AND BRAIN ENERGY 96

Role of Probiotics 97

Glucagon-like peptide 1 (GLP-1) hormone 98

VITAMINS FOR BLOOD GLUCOSE AND ENERGY METABOLISM 98

MINERALS FOR BLOOD GLUCOSE CONTROL 99

AMINO ACIDS AND BLOOD GLUCOSE REGULATION 101

L-Glutamine 101

Creatine 101

KEY TAKEAWAYS 103

CHAPTER 9: FASTING AND ITS IMPACT ON BRAIN HEALTH 105

UNDERSTANDING FASTING 105
FASTING AND BRAIN FUNCTION... 106
   Neuroprotective Impact.. 106
FASTING AND BLOOD GLUCOSE REGULATION 107
   Fasting as a Metabolic Reset 107
HOW TO FAST... 108
   Intermittent Fasting or Time-Restricted Eating 108
   Prolonged Fasting 109
   Personalized Responses to Fasting 110
   Practical Tips for Fasting... 111
KEY TAKEAWAYS 113

CHAPTER 10: OVERCOMING CHALLENGES AND STAYING MOTIVATED 115

STRESS MANAGEMENT AND BLOOD GLUCOSE CONTROL 115
HARNESSING TECHNOLOGY FOR HEALTH MANAGEMENT 118
CHECKLISTS FOR SUCCESS 118
   Creating a Personalized Action Plan 118
   Regular Review and Adaptation of the Plan 120
   Dealing with Setbacks and Maintaining Resilience.. 121
   Building Resilience and Staying Motivated... 121
   Social Support and Accountability 123
KEY TAKEAWAYS 124

CHAPTER 11: STAYING ON TOP OF BRAIN HEALTH 127

THE ROLE OF REGULAR HEALTH CHECK-UPS... 127
   Comprehensive Health Assessments for Preventive Care 127
   Collaborative Care Approach 128
BRAIN TRAINING AND COGNITIVE EXERCISES 128
   Cognitive Exercises for Brain Stimulation 129
   Adding Cognitive Activities to Your Daily Routine.. 130
KEY TAKEAWAYS 132

CONCLUSION.. 133

KEEPING THE KNOWLEDGE FLOWING 135

APPENDIX..**137**

BONUS: 12-WEEK CHALLENGE..**139**

PUTTING KNOWLEDGE INTO ACTION 139

Exercise 1: Keep a Food Diary 140

Exercise 2: Mindful Eating 141

Exercise 3: Brain-Boosting Meal Plan 142

Exercise 4: Label Reading Challenge...................................... 143

Exercise 5: Physical Activity Routine 144

Exercise 6: Stress Management Techniques 145

Exercise 7: Sleep Hygiene Checklist.. 146

Exercise 8: Blood Glucose Monitoring..................................... 148

Exercise 9: Hydration Challenge 148

Exercise 10: Brain-Boosting Recipe Swap 150

Exercise 11: Brain Training Games 151

Exercise 12: Staying Consistent Even When You Don't Want To 152

REFERENCES **161**

Introduction

Have you ever wondered about the hidden connection between what you eat and how your brain works? Your brain's performance is influenced by what you eat, how you eat it, and when you eat it. Ever heard someone say, "My brain feels a bit sluggish lately"? Get ready to connect the dots between how our brains work and the role of blood glucose.

This book is a guide to uncovering how blood glucose affects our thinking, and it's my privilege to be your companion on this exploration. I bring to this exploration over two decades of medical expertise as a physician and neurologist, blending the rigors of medical knowledge with the holistic principles of lifestyle medicine.

I was motivated to write this book as I often see the impact of blood sugar and metabolic health on brain health and wellbeing in my clinical practice. I am therefore writing this book with the mission of empowering people with high quality knowledge to take control of their health and wellbeing.

Join me as we dive into the details of how and why blood glucose plays a big role in our mental processes, and what you can do about it.

Objectives of This Book

I have written this book with these core objectives in mind:

1. **Understanding the brain-glucose connection:** This book will equip you with an understanding of how the brain-glucose

connection impacts our mental clarity and emotional well-being.

2. **Practical strategies for blood glucose management:** The book will arm you with tools—insights into dietary choices, lifestyle adjustments, and natural remedies—essential for mastering the management of blood glucose levels.

3. **Empowering you for better health and peak performance:** Beyond immediate gains, my goal is to empower you to take control of your long-term health, preventing conditions like insulin resistance, diabetes and their associated brain health problems, through well-informed choices.

The knowledge and skills you'll gain from this book will benefit you in the short-to-medium term, with actionable steps to feel better now, and also in years to come as you lay the foundation for long-term brain health benefits.

The Relevance of Blood Glucose and Brain Health

How is your blood glucose level relevant to your brain health? We will uncover this in the coming pages.

- **Impact on conditions like pre-diabetes, diabetes, and insulin resistance:** We will discuss how your body handles sugar, as well as sugar's role in insulin resistance, pre-diabetes, and diabetes. Understanding this connection empowers you to more effectively prevent and manage these conditions.
- **Connection to cognitive abilities:** Did you know that glucose is directly tied to cognitive function? Grasping this link empowers us to maximize cognitive sharpness from day to day, and to prevent cognitive decline. We'll be unlocking doors to both prevention and intervention.
- **Crucial role in mental health:** The ebb and flow of glucose can impact our mood and overall mental well-being. By

understanding this connection, we empower ourselves with more tools in our toolkit to foster mental resilience and well-being.

The book progresses through three general themes, each designed to equip you with essential knowledge and strategies for optimizing your brain health.

Theme 1: How Does It Work?

In Chapters 1 through 4, we'll cover how glucose in your body helps your brain work. We'll talk about how your body breaks down food to make glucose and how it travels to your brain to give it energy. You'll learn about insulin, a hormone that controls how much sugar is in your blood.

Theme 2: When Things Go Wrong

In Chapter 5, we'll talk about what happens when your blood sugar levels aren't right. We'll discuss how this can contribute to problems like diabetes, insulin resistance, and deteriorating vascular health, as well as the impact your sugar levels can have on your brain health and overall well-being.

Theme 3: What to Do About It

In Chapters 6 through 11, we'll offer practical tips to keep your blood sugar steady and your brain in top shape. We'll talk about things like what to eat, how to stay active, and ways to relax your mind. You'll find simple steps to follow that will help you stay healthy and feel good. Whether you're trying to avoid problems or deal with ones you already have, this section will give you the tools you need to take control of your health.

Within these pages, we'll guide you, step by step, on how to improve and protect your brain health. Consider this book your friendly companion, shedding light on how your brain works and helping you optimize your brain health.

Theme 1:

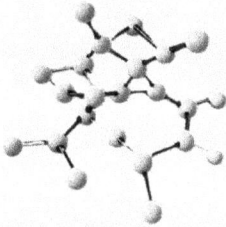

How does it work?

Chapter 1:
Understanding the Brain-Glucose Connection

Ever wondered why sometimes your brain feels like it's firing on all cylinders, and other times, it's a bit slow? Picture this: Your brain is like a finely tuned instrument, and the key to its melody lies in the delicate balance of glucose coursing through your bloodstream. Understanding the brain-glucose connection is not just about knowing what glucose is; it's about understanding how this sweet substance plays a crucial role in every mental note and thought. So, have you ever pondered the connection between glucose and your brain's performance?

The Basics of Brain Metabolism

Before we begin to explore the elaborate details of brain health, let's first establish a foundation by understanding the fundamentals of brain metabolism. This groundwork will equip us with the essential knowledge needed to dive into how our brains function and thrive.

Glucose as the Primary Fuel

Glucose, which comes from the breaking down of carbohydrates, is your brain's main energy source. It is the fuel that powers all the elaborate workings of the brain. To keep it working well, it's essential that the use of glucose be finely tuned.

If the energy balance in the brain gets disrupted, it sets the stage for various brain disorders (Mergenthaler et al., 2013). This can affect how well messages are sent in the brain, harm the networks of brain cells, and lead to conditions ranging from having trouble thinking to more severe disorders. Understanding this close relationship between glucose and the brain opens up opportunities for you to support your brain's health.

Brain Energy Consumption

Imagine the brain as a busy town within the human body, where every neuron is a bustling citizen engaged in various tasks. This activity requires a consistent and robust energy supply, much like the vibrant pulse of a city that never sleeps.

While the human brain constitutes a mere 2% of the body's overall weight, its energy demands are disproportionately high, consuming 20–25% of the body's glucose-derived energy. This energy is utilized for various functions, from regulating basic bodily processes to performing complex cognitive tasks (Mergenthaler et al., 2013). The substantial energy consumption reflects the constant need for the brain's cell signaling, cellular maintenance, and the sophisticated network of connections that govern our thoughts, emotions, and actions.

Brain Function and Glucose Dependency

The brain's heavy reliance on glucose is a strategic choice, shaped by its efficiency, speed, and precision of function. Glucose meets the formidable energy demands of this extraordinary organ.

Cognitive Performance and Glucose Levels

Metabolic switching and cognitive glucose sensitivity (CGS) are helpful concepts to understand as we explore how the brain manages changes in blood glucose levels. **Metabolic switching is the transition from glucose to fat as a source of energy, and CGS is the degree of glucose dependence for cognitive performance.** For example, a study involving cognitive tasks showed that sugar consumption after a 12-hour fast can temporarily improve cognitive function, especially in overweight men (Neukirchen et al., 2022). This example is to illustrate that the CGS in some people may lead them to sip on sugary drinks throughout the day when working on high cognitive tasks, but sadly this behavior inadvertently puts them at risk of diabetes.

Instead, the longer-term strategy is to improve metabolic flexibility.

Metabolic flexibility relates to the efficiency of metabolic switching, i.e. the body's ability to efficiently switch fuel sources between glucose and ketones, derived from the breakdown of fats. In this book, we will cover strategies for improving your metabolic flexibility through lifestyle choices, covered in Chapters 6-10.

Your Body's Blood Sugar Balancing Act

The hormones insulin and glucagon are important messengers that control the blood sugar levels in the body. They're like traffic directors, helping to manage the flow of sugar. The body carefully maintains a specific range of blood glucose levels to ensure optimal functioning.

When we eat, especially if we've had some sugary or starchy foods, our blood sugar goes up. Insulin steps in to guide that sugar into our cells, where it can be used for energy. It's like opening doors for sugar to get inside the cells.

When you haven't eaten for a while, maybe between meals or during the night, your blood sugar might start to drop. That's when glucagon steps in. It signals the liver to release stored sugar into the bloodstream. This helps keep our blood sugar from getting too low, making sure we have a steady supply of energy.

Our muscles also play a crucial role in maintaining blood sugar levels. They store glucose in the form of glycogen, which can be broken down into glucose by a hormone known as glucagon when needed.

The more muscle mass we have, the more efficient our bodies are at regulating blood sugar levels, as muscles are one of the primary sites for glucose disposal. Therefore, maintaining muscle through regular exercise and a balanced diet is essential for overall blood glucose control, which we'll cover in greater depth in upcoming chapters on lifestyle modifications.

The control of appetite is closely linked to changes in glucose levels after meals, with the brain playing a role here in managing hunger and satiety.

The brain quickly adapts in response to fluctuations in blood glucose levels, maintaining essential tasks despite changes in energy availability.

When fasting or following a low-carbohydrate diet, the brain can utilize ketones as an alternative energy source when glucose levels are low. Ketones, derived from fat breakdown in the liver, serve as a vital backup fuel for the brain during times of glucose scarcity.

However, disruptions in glucose control mechanisms can lead to various health issues, affecting both physical and mental well-being. These topics will be further explored in Chapter 4.

Glucose Sensing in the Brain

Glucose sensing refers to the ability of cells, particularly neurons in the brain, to detect changes in the concentration of glucose (sugar) in the bloodstream. This sensing mechanism allows cells to monitor and respond to fluctuations in glucose levels, which is important for maintaining metabolic balance and regulating various physiological processes such as energy metabolism, appetite, and hormonal signaling. Let's take a quick look at how your body stays on top of this process.

- The brain's role in regulating glucose levels is managed by a specialized region called the hypothalamus and the brainstem, that actively monitor changes in blood sugar levels.

- Glucose transporters, are special proteins called GLUTs, that help sugar enter brain cells.

- Once absorbed, glucose undergoes metabolic processes to release energy vital for neuronal function.

- These metabolic activities influence the electrical signals within the neurons.

- Changes in electrical activity prompt the release of neurotransmitters, facilitating communication between neurons.

- The hypothalamus integrates signals from glucose-sensing neurons with information from other body parts. This integration allows the brain to regulate essential functions such as appetite, energy expenditure, and hormonal signals.

This regulatory process helps maintain metabolic balance within the body. And the brain's active involvement here in managing glucose levels, ensures optimal conditions for sustained cognitive function.

Blood-Brain Barrier Integrity and Glucose Levels

The blood-brain barrier acts as a vigilant guardian of your brain, selectively allowing essential nutrients and molecules to enter, while preventing potentially harmful substances from passing through.

Glucose plays a key role in maintaining this equilibrium. Fluctuations in glucose levels can influence the integrity of the blood-brain barrier's structure and function in two main ways.

Firstly, specialized proteins known as glucose transporters allow the passage of glucose from the bloodstream into the brain. Altered glucose levels can disrupt the regulation of these transporters.

Secondly, altered glucose metabolism can trigger inflammatory cascades that disrupt the tight junctions between cells that make up the barrier.

As a result of increased permeability of the blood-brain barrier, substances that are typically restricted may enter the brain, risking neuroinflammation.

The interplay between glucose metabolism, blood-brain barrier integrity, and neuronal health has important implications for cognitive function. Changes in glucose levels, if not regulated effectively, may contribute to cognitive decline, emphasizing the importance of maintaining stable glucose levels for long-term brain health.

Key Takeaways

In our first chapter, we discovered some exciting facts about how your brain and blood sugar work together.

- Blood glucose is the brain's preferred energy source, consuming 20-25% of the body's derived energy despite only constituting 2% of body weight.

- The body maintains blood sugar balance through hormones like insulin and glucagon, with lifestyle factors playing a crucial role in glucose regulation.

- When you're not eating, your brain efficiently utilizes its energy, ensuring you can keep thinking even with limited sugar available.

- Metabolic flexibility is the ability to easily switch between glucose and fat for energy, and an important concept in understanding how glucose levels affect cognitive performance. It is influenced by lifestyle factors which we cover in subsequent chapters.

- Maintaining a steady blood glucose level is vital for optimal brain function.

- Stable blood glucose helps protect the brain by maintaining the blood-brain barrier, which guards against inflammation and supports long-term brain health.

***

Next, in Chapter 2, we'll continue with a deeper dive into how your blood sugar influences your brain functions.

Chapter 2:
Into the Brain Cells

Once glucose is produced, it enters the bloodstream, and the body can then use it to produce energy. In this chapter, we delve into the neurobiology of how brain cells use glucose.

Neurobiology of Glucose Metabolism

Within the brain, neurons and astrocytes work together in a coordinated manner to absorb glucose. Neurons are often referred to as the brain's information messengers. They are specialized cells responsible for transmitting signals throughout the nervous system. Picture them as the conductors of this amazing choir, directing the flow of information within the brain.

Astrocytes, on the other hand, are star-shaped cells that provide crucial support to neurons. Think of them as the backstage crew ensuring the smooth operation of the entire cognitive performance. Among their many functions, astrocytes play a pivotal role in regulating the brain's environment and assisting neurons in times of increased demand.

In Chapter 1, we explored the role of the blood-brain barrier and understood that it only lets important things, like glucose, pass through.

Let's imagine glucose transporters (GLUT) as the bouncers at a VIP entrance. They hold the key to unlock the door, ensuring that only glucose, the brain's preferred fuel, gets inside. This controlled process maintains the brain's energy levels just right, akin to regulating access to a VIP area.

Neurons and astrocytes possess specialized mechanisms to capture glucose from the bloodstream.

Neurons are the primary consumers of glucose, and actively transport it across their cell membranes. This process is vital for the production of adenosine triphosphate (ATP), the cellular energy currency that fuels the activities of neurons.

Astrocytes, which act like helper brain cells, also use glucose. They help move a steady and regulated supply of glucose from the bloodstream to neurons. Astrocytes also convert a portion of glucose into lactate, an additional energy source for neurons when they are very active (Beard et al., 2021).

Glucose Metabolism Pathways

After glucose has been taken up by these brain cells, it is broken down further through two pathways: glycolysis and oxidative phosphorylation. These pathways create ATP, the energy currency that fuels all the brain's activities.

Now let's take a deeper dive into these two main steps: glycolysis and oxidative phosphorylation.

Glycolysis starts the breakdown of glucose into smaller molecules, releasing a modest amount of energy. Think of it as the first spark that sets the stage for a more significant energy production performance.

Now, let's break down the key steps in this pathway (Harris & Harper, 2015):

1. **Glucose Entry:** Glucose, the primary player, enters the glycolytic pathway.

2. **Energy Investment:** Initially, a bit of energy is used to prepare glucose for the subsequent stages.

3. **Splitting Glucose:** Glucose is split into two smaller molecules, creating a pair of three-carbon compounds.

4. **Energy Release:** In this step, a modest amount of energy is released, akin to a small burst of power.

5. **Formation of ATP:** Some of this released energy is used to produce a few ATP molecules.

6. **Creating Pyruvate:** The three-carbon compounds are further processed, ultimately forming pyruvate.

Glycolysis only produces a small amount of energy. But it's important because it sets up the second step that makes more energy: oxidative phosphorylation.

Oxidative phosphorylation unfolds within the mitochondria, which are like little powerhouses inside your cells. Through a series of steps, molecules generated from glycolysis enter the mitochondria, to create energy in the form of ATP (Deshpande & Mohiuddin, 2020), as follows:

1. **Mitochondrial Entry:** The molecules produced in glycolysis move into the mitochondria.

2. **Citric Acid Cycle (Krebs Cycle):** The journey kicks off with the citric acid cycle, a series of chemical reactions that further break down the molecules, extracting a bit more energy.

3. **Electron Transport Chain:** This is the highlight of the show. High-energy electrons generated in the previous steps move through a series of proteins in the inner mitochondrial membrane. As they travel, energy is released and used to pump charge particles, called protons, across the membrane.

4. **ATP Synthesis:** The pumped protons create an energy gradient. The protons flow back across the mitochondrial membrane, through a protein called ATP synthase. This creates ATP for your brain.

5. **Oxygen's Crucial Role:** Oxygen plays a vital role in this process, serving as the ultimate electron acceptor. It ensures the smooth flow of electrons through the entire chain.

Mitochondrial Role in Glucose Metabolism

In your brain's busy world, mitochondria are like little factories working hard to turn glucose into ATP, the energy currency that your brain needs. These mitochondria are tiny assembly lines where glucose goes through a set of steps. As we just covered, each part of the mitochondria has its own job, like different workstations, making sure glucose becomes ATP.

This whole process is a well-organized system, providing a constant supply of ATP to keep your brain's energy flowing smoothly. The role of mitochondria in handling glucose is vital, ensuring your brain stays lively and active in everything it does.

Even though mitochondria are important energy makers in brain cells, they can sometimes have problems. These problems can harm how the brain normally works. This includes conditions where damaged mitochondria contribute to the development of neurodegenerative diseases. Problems with mitochondria—such as membrane leakage, electrolyte imbalances, activation of pathways that lead to cell death, and the removal of damaged mitochondria—have been connected to the development of diseases like Alzheimer's, Parkinson's, Huntington's, and ischemic stroke (Norat et al., 2020).

Brain Energy Demands

The brain is like the rest of the body, where different types of activities need different amounts of energy, depending on the task and how intense it is.

Resting vs. Active Brain Glucose Needs

When your brain is at rest, quietly overseeing essential functions like maintaining bodily functions and sustaining basic awareness, it needs less glucose. During this phase, the brain operates on a more conservative energy budget, like a dimly lit room requiring less power.

Conversely, when your brain transitions into a state of activity like engaging in cognitive tasks, the demand for glucose rises dramatically. This requires a substantial influx of glucose to fuel the increased energy demands, allowing the brain to operate optimally.

Cognitive Demands and Glucose Metabolism

During demanding cognitive tasks, specific brain regions intensify their glucose consumption. Imaging techniques like functional magnetic resonance imaging (fMRI) reveal increased glucose use in areas such as the prefrontal cortex and hippocampus, which are centers for cognition, memory, and learning. As mental tasks become more challenging, the brain strategically allocates resources, with glucose consumption mirroring the complexity of the task at hand.

Sustained mental efforts require heightened neural activity, leading to increased glucose demand to support concentration, information processing, and complex cognitive functions. During continued mental tasks, there is an increased demand for energy, particularly in the prefrontal cortex. Depleted glucose levels in this area may result in mental fatigue, decreased alertness, and impaired decision-making. **Thus, maintaining stable blood glucose levels is important for optimal brain function during extended periods of cognitive focus.**

Glucose, Oxidative Stress, and Brain Health

Let's now talk about reactive oxygen species (ROS). We covered that mitochondria are like the powerhouses of the cell, generating energy currency in the form of ATP. Mitochondria produce ROS as natural byproducts when turning glucose into energy. However, this process has consequences (Liemburg-Apers et al., 2015).

ROS include molecules like superoxide and hydrogen peroxide, which are highly reactive compounds. When produced in excess, they lead to oxidative stress. The balance between ROS production and oxidative stress is critical for the optimal health of the cell.

Fluctuations in glucose levels can cause an imbalance of ROS production by the mitochondria. When we have an excess of glucose, like when we consume a lot of sugary or carbohydrate-rich foods, the mitochondria might end up working overtime. This can lead to an increased production of ROS.

Excessive oxidative stress can cause damage to cellular components, including proteins, lipids, and DNA, and is believed to play a role in neurodegenerative diseases.

Mitochondrial Antioxidant Defense

The mitochondria have a remarkable defense system to shield themselves and your brain cells from potential harm caused by oxidative stress, especially when glucose levels fluctuate. Within the mitochondria, there are enzymes and molecules that act like internal guardians, countering the effects of ROS. These defenders play a crucial role in maintaining a balanced environment and preventing excessive damage.

One of the key players in this defense mechanism is an enzyme called superoxide dismutase, which acts as a scavenger, neutralizing harmful ROS (Jena et al., 2023). Another essential component is glutathione, a molecule that helps recycle and neutralize ROS, acting like a cellular janitor that keeps the internal environment tidy.

Under varying glucose conditions, these defense mechanisms adapt and adjust their activity. When glucose levels are high, indicating an influx of energy production, these mitochondrial defenders kick into high gear to manage the potential increase in ROS. Conversely, during periods of low glucose, they stay vigilant in the background, ensuring a consistent defense against any oxidative stress that might arise.

Think of it as a dynamic security system within your cells, always ready to respond and adapt to changing conditions. This ensures the protection of your mitochondria and, consequently, the well-being of your brain cells.

Antioxidant Defense Mechanisms in the Brain

Within the brain, there is also a robust network of natural defense mechanisms to counteract oxidative stress arising from glucose metabolism. Enzymes with antioxidant properties, such as catalase and peroxidase, act as powerful guardians within brain cells. They target and neutralize harmful reactive molecules, preventing them from causing damage to vital cellular structures. Neurons themselves possess built-in mechanisms to fight oxidative stress, and astrocytes, which support the neurons, also act as scavengers of ROS.

Just like the mitochondrial's antioxidant defense, the brain's antioxidant defense mechanisms are not static; they adapt according to demands of varying glucose levels. During periods of increased glucose metabolism, these defenses intensify to manage the potential rise in oxidative stress. Conversely, when glucose availability is limited, the brain's antioxidant machinery remains active in the background, providing continuous protection against potential damage.

Ketones vs. Glucose: Alternative Brain Fuels

Although glucose is the major player in the brain's energy game, it's not the only contender. Ketones, derived from the breakdown of fats, are an alternative fuel source that the brain can also use.

During periods of low glucose availability, such as fasting or adherence to a ketogenic diet, the body undergoes a metabolic shift. In response to reduced glucose levels, the liver produces ketones to provide energy to the brain.

In this ketogenic state, the brain switches its primary energy preference from glucose to ketones. Ketones become a valuable substitute, sustaining the brain's energy needs even when glucose availability is limited. Some people even report improved mental clarity and focus when their brain has adapted to using ketones (Altayyar et al., 2022).

This metabolic flexibility reflects the brain's remarkable ability to maintain functionality under varying nutritional conditions. We mentioned the benefit of improving this metabolic flexibility in the Chapter 1. Throughout this book, we'll cover lifestyle measures that can enhance your ability to adjust to these different fuel sources.

Comparison of Ketones and Glucose

One key aspect of comparing ketones and glucose is in the efficiency of energy production. Ketones have the advantage of being more energy efficient. When metabolized, ketones generate more ATP per unit of oxygen consumed compared to glucose. This heightened efficiency suggests that, pound for pound, ketones could potentially provide more energy to the brain.

The story doesn't end with efficiency. Emerging research suggests potential neuroprotective effects associated with ketone metabolism. These include cellular resilience and defense against oxidative stress (Yang et al., 2019).

The ketogenic diet, designed to induce a state of ketosis, has been shown to reduce seizure frequency in some individuals with epilepsy. Additionally, in conditions where glucose metabolism in the brain is impaired, ketones can be a promising source of alternative energy. For example, in research on Alzheimer's disease, ketones can potentially serve as a supplementary energy source for brain cells, in situations of compromised glucose utilization (Ramezani et al., 2023).

Key Takeaways

In this chapter, we explored how your brain uses glucose and ketones for energy, and the role of the mitochondria in energy production. Here are the key takeaways:

- Glucose is the brain's primary fuel, but it's not the only option. Ketones, derived from fat breakdown, can serve as an alternative energy source.

- Glucose metabolism involves two main pathways: glycolysis and oxidative phosphorylation. Glycolysis starts the breakdown process, while oxidative phosphorylation, occurring in mitochondria, produces most of the brain's energy (ATP).

- Mitochondria are like tiny powerhouses in brain cells, converting glucose into ATP, the energy currency that fuels the brain.

- The brain's energy needs vary depending on its activity. Resting states require less glucose, while demanding cognitive tasks increase energy consumption in specific brain regions.

- The brain has natural defense mechanisms against oxidative stress, which can occur during energy production. These defenses adapt to changing glucose levels, helping to protect brain cells.

**

These insights underscore the importance of maintaining stable blood sugar levels and improving your metabolic flexibility. In Chapter 3, we'll dive into the world of blood sugar issues. Let's uncover ways to identify the imbalances in your blood sugar and understand what they mean.

Chapter 3:
Identifying Blood Glucose Imbalances

Blood glucose imbalances can have a powerful impact on your overall health and well-being. When blood glucose control is affected, it can lead to several health conditions.

Diabetes is a condition where blood sugar levels are persistently high. You may be surprised to know that in 2015, it was estimated that 30.2 million Americans have diabetes, but 24% hadn't been officially diagnosed (Chia et al., 2018). This means around 7.2 million Americans unknowingly have a negative health impact from undiagnosed (and untreated) diabetes. That's quite shocking. An absence of diagnosis simply means that the person isn't receiving the correct treatment to manage and care for their condition, potentially resulting in more health problems.

However, regardless of whether you have diabetes or not, your overall health can benefit from understanding how your blood glucose levels work and what occurs. In this chapter, we will cover how to identify blood glucose imbalances.

Understanding Glycemic Variability

First, let's take a moment to understand glycemic variability. This refers to the fluctuations of your blood sugar levels throughout the day.

These fluctuations play a significant role in influencing various aspects of your mental well-being. For instance, when blood sugar levels drop, you might experience shifts in mood, such as irritability or feeling low on energy. It's like the dimming of a light when the power source isn't steady. Similarly, your cognition may be impacted, leading to difficulties with concentration or memory recall.

On the other hand, maintaining a steady supply of glucose ensures that your brain operates with optimal mental clarity. It's like providing the ideal conditions for a well-lit and smoothly functioning room. When blood sugar levels are stable, your brain can perform cognitive tasks more efficiently, enhancing your ability to focus, solve problems, and retain information.

Factors Influencing Glycemic Variability

A number of factors affect glycemic variability. Your food choices, how active you are, your stress levels, sleep, and even hormonal changes all contribute to the rhythm of your blood glucose. Understanding these elements gives you the power to fine-tune your blood sugar balance. We'll do a deeper dive into these factors, and how you can improve them, in chapters 6 and 7.

Glycemic Variability and Health Outcomes

Research has established a strong link between glycemic variability and health outcomes, particularly in the context of diabetes (Kota et al., 2013). High glycemic variability can contribute to insulin resistance, as frequent spikes and crashes in blood sugar levels may reduce cells' responsiveness to insulin, the hormone regulating blood glucose. These fluctuations may bring about complications associated with diabetes, increasing the risk of conditions like heart disease, kidney problems, and neuropathy due to damage to blood vessels, nerves, and organs.

Frequent fluctuations in blood glucose levels may also contribute to inflammation and impair the function of the endothelium, the inner lining of blood vessels. Endothelial dysfunction is a key factor in the development of atherosclerosis, a condition where arteries become narrowed and hardened, increasing the risk of heart disease.

Additionally, fluctuating glucose levels also have the potential to elevate your cholesterol levels.

Unstable blood glucose levels can lead to fluctuations in blood pressure (Sezer et al., 2020). These fluctuations, especially if they are frequent, may strain the cardiovascular system. Long-term exposure to high blood pressure increases the risk of heart disease and stroke.

If blood glucose levels were to remain consistently high (a condition known as hyperglycemia), it could lead to the formation of advanced glycation end-products (AGEs). These AGEs can contribute to various complications, such as damage to blood vessels, nerves, and tissues, impacting organs like the kidneys, eyes, and heart.

On the other hand, if blood glucose levels stayed consistently low (hypoglycemia), it would deprive the brain and other vital organs of the energy they need, potentially causing symptoms like confusion, dizziness, and, in severe cases, unconsciousness. Therefore, the body's precise regulation of blood glucose is crucial for maintaining overall health and preventing potential complications.

Recognizing this connection is essential to grasping the broader picture of overall health. It's about understanding how variability in blood sugar levels contributes to various health aspects beyond just one specific condition. In Chapter 6, we'll discover strategies on how to monitor and manage glycemic variability.

Hypoglycemia: Causes and Symptoms

Hypoglycemia is when the level of glucose in your blood drops to a point that is lower than normal. Like many health conditions, this can occur as a result of the lifestyles we lead. The following are some potential causes:

- **Missing meals:** Erratic skipping of meals may disrupt the regular supply of glucose needed for bodily functions. When this happens, the body may lack the carbohydrates necessary to maintain blood glucose levels in some susceptible individuals.

The erratic skipping of meals can be considered differently from fasting, and in Chapter 8, we will discuss this in detail.

- **Excessive exercise:** Physical activity increases the body's demand for energy, primarily sourced from glucose. During intense or prolonged exercise, the muscles use more glucose to meet energy requirements. Without sufficient replenishment through food, this increased demand can result in lower blood glucose levels. Balancing exercise with proper nutrition is key to preventing hypoglycemia associated with excessive physical activity.

- **Insulin overdose in diabetic patients:** For individuals with diabetes, insulin is commonly used to manage blood sugar levels. However, an overdose of insulin can lead to a rapid drop in blood glucose levels, causing hypoglycemia. It's critical for individuals with diabetes to carefully adhere to prescribed insulin doses, monitor blood sugar levels regularly, and coordinate adjustments with healthcare providers to avoid the risk of hypoglycemia.

Symptoms and Immediate Management

When your body's blood sugar drops too low, it may create a stress response, which could include symptoms of shakiness, dizziness, or cold sweats. For people with diabetes who receive insulin injections, as hypoglycemia intensifies, it can progress to severe symptoms such as confusion or, in extreme cases, loss of consciousness.

A proactive approach to preventing hypoglycemia is to consider the timing of your meals and your food choices to stabilize your blood sugar.

Recurrent hypoglycemia is characterized by repeated low blood sugar levels that occur frequently and could have a negative impact on the brain, contributing to cognitive issues. This prolonged stress can also contribute to cardiovascular complications, affecting the health of your heart over the long term.

Hyperglycemia: Recognizing the Warning Signs

Hyperglycemia, or having too much sugar in the blood, occurs when blood sugar levels rise above normal. It can lead to symptoms such as increased thirst and frequent urination as the body attempts to eliminate the excess sugar. These signs may indicate the onset of diabetes, and they can be accompanied by fatigue and blurred vision. Recognizing these early signals is crucial for maintaining overall health and well-being.

Consistently high blood sugar levels can lead to diabetic retinopathy, causing damage to the blood vessels in the eyes and potentially leading to vision problems or blindness. Additionally, chronic hyperglycemia can result in neuropathy, affecting nerve function and causing symptoms such as numbness, tingling, or pain, especially in the extremities.

Hyperglycemia in Non-Diabetics

Even if you don't have diabetes, your blood sugar can sometimes go up, especially during stressful times. This is called stress-induced hyperglycemia. In a stressful situation—it could be an exam, a work deadline, or any other challenging scenario—your body's stress response kicks in, triggering the release of hormones like cortisol and adrenaline. These hormones prepare your body for a 'fight or flight' response.

Here's where the blood sugar connection comes into play. The hormones released during stress signal to your liver to release more glucose into the bloodstream, providing a quick energy boost to cope with the perceived threat. It's your body's way of gearing up for action, ensuring you have the fuel needed to confront or escape a stressful situation.

In the short term, this increase in blood sugar is a normal and adaptive response. Your body is designed to handle occasional stress, and this mechanism helps you perform better in challenging situations. However, problems arise when stress becomes chronic or frequent.

If stress-induced hyperglycemia happens too often, it can strain your body's insulin response, potentially leading to insulin resistance over time. Insulin is a hormone that helps cells absorb glucose from the bloodstream. When the body becomes less responsive to insulin, it can result in persistently elevated blood sugar levels, a precursor to type 2 diabetes.

So, while stress-induced hyperglycemia is natural and temporary, it's essential to manage chronic stress to prevent potential long-term health issues. It's a survival strategy that's beneficial in moderation but warrants attention if it becomes a frequent occurrence.

Metabolic Health

Metabolic syndrome is a combination of health conditions that collaborate to increase the risk of heart disease, stroke, and diabetes. These conditions include increased blood pressure, high blood sugar, excess body fat surrounding internal organs (around the waist), and abnormal cholesterol or triglyceride levels. To diagnose metabolic syndrome, specific criteria are used, such as measuring waist circumference, checking fasting glucose and insulin levels, examining lipid profiles, and taking blood pressure measurements.

When these conditions collectively surpass certain thresholds, they are identified as metabolic syndrome. Understanding and monitoring these factors serves as a compass, guiding individuals away from potential health risks and toward a path of improved well-being.

Navigating Insulin Resistance and Metabolic Health

The metabolism acts as your body's energy system. Since energy is required for all bodily processes and activities, it makes sense that your metabolic health is crucial to your overall health and well-being. Like most systems within your body, an imbalance in the energy system can trigger health problems.

Insulin resistance is a condition with the power to trigger an imbalance in the body's energy metabolism, impacting your overall metabolic health. But what is insulin resistance? This happens when your body is unable to respond effectively to insulin—a hormone we now know contributes to your metabolic function.

When this happens, your body will overcompensate by producing even more insulin, triggering a state known as hyperinsulinemia. In this state, several metabolic consequences may occur, including high blood pressure, elevated blood sugar levels, abnormal cholesterol levels, increased inflammation, and a higher risk of blood clots. And these conditions could then lead to further negative effects.

Insulin resistance can be a precursor to health conditions like type 2 diabetes. It's even believed that insulin resistance might precede the development of this health condition by 10 to 15 years (Freeman & Pennings, 2019). This means that preventing insulin resistance could help delay or stop the onset of type 2 diabetes. But how do you do this?

Waist circumference has been used as an easy way to detect the possible onset of insulin resistance. If your waist's circumference is more than half of your body height, you may have—or be at a higher risk of—insulin resistance.

Fortunately, preventing insulin resistance can be as easy as making use of lifestyle interventions. Participate in regular physical activity, maintain a healthy diet, and manage your weight effectively. In later chapters, we'll take a closer look at how such activities could help you manage your health and protect you from insulin resistance. If you have an existing health condition, then you may need to consult your healthcare provider before making changes or taking up a new physical activity or diet.

It's recommended that you attend frequent health checkups with your healthcare provider, especially if you're concerned about insulin resistance. During the checkup, your healthcare provider can assess your blood pressure, blood sugar, cholesterol levels, and stress levels. If your family has a history of diabetes, be sure to mention this to your provider so that you can take proactive measures to care for your health and delay or prevent the onset of this condition.

Before we move on to the next section, reflect on what you've learned and remember that your continued health is worth the effort it takes to maintain it. Understanding how your blood glucose is tested can also help you make informed decisions when discussing your health during a checkup.

Blood Glucose Testing Methods

It's important to regularly have your glucose levels checked, and this can be done as part of your health check with your doctor or healthcare practitioner. This allows you to monitor your health in a better way and gives you a chance to manage any situation that could arise before it gets out of hand.

There is a range of blood glucose testing methods available, spanning from traditional to cutting-edge techniques. Let's begin by exploring the traditional finger-prick tests. This method involves a small needle prick to your finger, drawing a drop of blood. The blood is then applied to a test strip, and a glucose meter reads the concentration, providing a quick snapshot of your current blood glucose level. This gives reliable results, but you need to stop and check your blood at that moment. It's a bit of a pause in your day.

Continuous glucose monitoring is another way to track blood glucose levels throughout the day. A specialized device, known as a continuous glucose monitor (CGM), uses a sensor that is inserted into the skin to measure glucose levels.

The sensor then measures the levels of glucose in the fluid found between your cells, and this data is stored on your smartphone where it can be shared with your healthcare provider. Continuous glucose monitoring is generally used by individuals who suffer from type 1 or type 2 diabetes.

That's because a CGM can continuously measure blood glucose levels, allowing you to understand how these levels change and what might be affecting them. Such information is valuable in helping you make informed decisions about the food and drinks you consume, the medications you take, and the level of activity you participate in so that you can keep your blood glucose levels within their safe target range.

For a broader view, there are tests like the oral glucose tolerance test (OGTT) and the hemoglobin A1c test. OGTT involves fasting and consuming a glucose solution to track the body's response, while hemoglobin A1c offers a longer-term perspective by measuring average glucose levels over three months.

There's also the historical method of urine glucose testing, which identifies glucose presence in urine as an indication of elevated blood sugar. Each method contributes to a comprehensive understanding of blood glucose levels and plays a crucial role in managing one's health.

Interestingly, there may be emerging Artificial Intelligence technology that provide people with personalized recommendations for managing their blood glucose levels. As research and innovation continue, we can anticipate even more breakthroughs, making blood sugar monitoring not just efficient but also smarter and tailored to individual needs.

Key Takeaways

In this chapter, we learned about spotting issues with our blood sugar levels. Here are some important points to remember:

- Think of your blood sugar level as a steady stream. Fluctuations can affect your mood, energy, and cognitive abilities. Stable glucose levels provide optimal conditions for clear thinking and focus.

- Your diet, physical activity, stress levels, and sleep, all contribute to the rhythm of your blood glucose. Understanding these factors empowers you to manage and fine-tune your daily health.

- Research shows a strong link between glycemic variability and health, especially in diabetes. High variability can lead to insulin resistance and is associated with complications like heart disease, kidney problems, and neuropathy.

- Maintaining good metabolic health is vital for both our bodies and our brains. This involves addressing insulin resistance and taking proactive steps to prevent or improve metabolic health through lifestyle changes.

***

Next up, Chapter 4 takes us into the connection between how we feel and the sugar in our blood. We'll discover how keeping our blood sugar in check is not only important for our body but is also crucial for our mood and mental health.

Chapter 4:
Mental Health, Mood, and Blood Glucose

Do you know the broader impact of blood sugar extends beyond just energy levels? What if it could influence your mood, mental well-being, and even your daily experiences?

It's worth recognizing the profound impact that post-meal blood sugar fluctuations can exert on our overall mood and well-being over time. Research suggests the consumption of sugary foods and beverages may not only contribute to immediate fluctuations in blood glucose levels but could also have long-term implications for mental health.

Blood Glucose and Emotional Regulation

You know how on some days, you can feel on top of the world, while on others, not so much? Well, it turns out your blood sugar might have something to do with it (Kay, 2019). In this chapter, we're diving into the science of how your glucose levels can play a role in your mood and emotional stability.

Within your body, the brain and the endocrine system work in tandem to regulate various functions, including your mood. When blood glucose levels fluctuate, it triggers a cascade of events, starting with your neurotransmitters, which are chemicals that transmit signals between nerve cells. The primary neurotransmitters affected include serotonin, dopamine, and norepinephrine, which play pivotal roles in regulating mood and emotional responses. Changes in blood glucose levels can impact their synthesis, release, and reuptake, leading to alterations in mood.

Simultaneously, insulin plays a significant role in emotional regulation. By facilitating the absorption of glucose into cells from the bloodstream, insulin ensures a steady supply of fuel for cellular activities, including those involved in maintaining emotional stability and mood regulation.

Moreover, hormonal balance, including the release of stress hormones like cortisol, is connected to your blood glucose. Fluctuations can influence the secretion of these hormones, contributing to emotional responses and stability.

But here's the big reveal: **Irregular blood sugar isn't just about feeling a bit off.** It can actually be linked to serious mood disorders. Research has established correlations between irregular blood glucose levels and conditions such as anxiety and bipolar disorder. These connections underline the relationship between the body's glucose regulation and mental health (Calkin et al., 2013).

In the case of anxiety, fluctuations in blood glucose contribute to heightened feelings of unease and restlessness. For bipolar disorder, characterized by extreme mood swings between manic and depressive states, irregular blood glucose levels could potentially play a role in intensifying these episodes.

Nurturing Emotional Resilience through Balanced Blood Glucose

Understanding the vital connection between blood glucose and emotional well-being opens the door to empowering strategies. By adopting mindful dietary choices and making simple lifestyle adjustments, you hold the key to fostering emotional stability. These are covered in depth in the second half of this book.

Blood Sugar Balance and Stress Response

The relationship between blood sugar balance and the body's stress response gives us essential insight into our overall well-being. The hypothalamic-pituitary-adrenal (HPA) axis is a key player in the body's stress response system. In situations of blood sugar imbalance, especially in conditions like pre-diabetes and type 2 diabetes, the HPA axis can experience altered function.

But what is the HPA axis?

- The **hypothalamus** is your brain's control center that senses stress and signals the next steps.

- The **pituitary gland** releases hormones that instruct other glands, especially the adrenal glands.

- The **adrenal glands** pump out stress hormones, including cortisol, responding to the pituitary's cue.

As such, altered functioning of the HPA axis can negatively impact our overall well-being. This could result in additional problems, like an increased susceptibility to depression. Beyond mental health, disruptions to this axis may trigger downstream effects like increased gluconeogenesis (glucose production) and dyslipidemia (abnormal lipid levels).

Stress also acts as an additional trigger and further activates the HPA axis, heightening the stress response and releasing stress hormones such as cortisol. The stress response is a normal process in the body, but problems may emerge when stress becomes persistent and chronic. Here's a quick look at what happens inside your body when you experience chronic stress:

- Stress initiates hormonal surges, prompting the liver to release more glucose into the bloodstream to meet increased energy demands.

- Elevated blood sugar levels result from this heightened release of glucose

- Insulin release attempts to regulate blood sugar, but excessive stress can diminish insulin's effectiveness, reducing its efficiency.

- High blood sugar exacerbates stress symptoms, leading to mood swings, irritability, and overall unease, intensifying the stress response.

- This creates a cyclical pattern: Stress influences blood sugar, and blood sugar impacts stress, forming a continuous loop that can escalate if left unaddressed.

In the coming chapters, we cover lifestyle strategies to help you break this cycle, including sleep, nutrition, exercise and more.

Dietary Sugars and Depression

Remember that while sugar is found in candy, pasta, bread, and baked goods, it's also found in vegetables, grains, and fruits. In other words, even if you aren't actively adding sugar to your food, you're most likely consuming sugar. So how could this impact your mood?

Depending on the foods you eat, the type of sugar you ingest can have different effects on your mind and body. For example, natural sugars found in fruits and vegetables are less likely to impact your mental health or mood, and they are less likely to contribute to additional health problems like increased inflammation. Additionally, fruits and vegetables contain phytonutrients that are anti-oxidants, protecting your mitochondria and brain cells. Processed sugars, however, like those found in candy and refined carbohydrates, often contribute to poor mental health and mood disorders because of their ability to trigger inflammation throughout your body—and because of the addictive nature of these types of sugar.

Sugar can be considered to have addictive qualities because of its ability to interact with your brain and stimulate its reward center. This means that eating sugar brings you pleasure. So, whenever you feel a negative emotion, like stress or sadness, you may reach for a sugary food to help you feel better. When this becomes a habit, you may find yourself feeling irritable or angry when you don't consume sugar, and this is in addition to the negative emotions you may already be experiencing. But what happens in your body when you ingest sugar?

When we consume high amounts of processed sugars, our body experiences a rapid spike in blood glucose levels. In response, the pancreas releases insulin to help cells absorb and use this excess glucose for energy. However, this rapid surge in blood sugar is frequently followed by a swift decline, resulting in a condition often referred to as *reactive hypoglycemia*. It's worth noting that, while it might not precisely meet the medical criteria for hypoglycemia based on blood glucose recordings, the speed of this reduction might be able to trigger symptoms that are similar to hypoglycemia.

This perspective is based on my own experiences and observations in my clinical practice. It has led me to investigate how non-diabetic patients experience the symptoms associated with this rapid drop in blood sugar levels through continuous glucose monitoring. Interestingly, I've discovered that adopting specific lifestyle strategies—like the ones discussed in this book—can help stabilize this type of blood sugar fluctuation.

Keep in mind that the fluctuation in blood sugar levels can trigger various physiological responses. The body perceives the rapid drop in glucose as a stressor, prompting the release of stress hormones such as cortisol and adrenaline. These hormonal shifts can impact the neurotransmitters in the brain, including serotonin, which plays a crucial role in regulating mood.

While it's okay to treat ourselves now and then, it's important to remember that too much sugar might not be great for our mood. Eating a mix of different foods with important nutrients for our bodies can help keep both our physical and mental health in check. And if you wish to consume a sweet item, consider having this after a balanced meal to avoid the sugar spikes and crashes.

Sugar Consumption and Inflammation

When we consume excessive amounts of sugar, especially in the form of processed and refined sugars found in various foods, it can trigger an inflammatory response in the body (Ma et al., 2022). This process involves the release of inflammatory molecules, such as cytokines, as the body reacts to the perceived threat posed by the sudden surge in sugar.

Chronic and excessive sugar intake can lead to prolonged inflammation, a state often referred to as systemic inflammation. This inflammation doesn't just affect a specific part of the body; it can become a widespread and persistent condition. In the context of mental health, this systemic inflammation may have implications for the brain.

The brain is particularly sensitive to inflammation, and studies have suggested that chronic inflammation may contribute to the development and progression of mental health conditions, including depression (Lee & Giuliani, 2019). Inflammation can affect the balance of neurotransmitters, disrupt neural circuits, and influence the function of brain regions associated with mood regulation.

Therefore, the link between sugar consumption and inflammation becomes a noteworthy factor in understanding how dietary choices may impact mental health. Reducing your intake of sugary foods may contribute to managing inflammation and, consequently, support better mental well-being, especially for those susceptible to or dealing with depression.

Impact on Gut Microbiome

Let's unravel the impact of a high-sugar diet on the gut microbiome, something that plays a crucial role in our mental well-being. Your gut microbiome is a bustling community of tiny organisms, each with a specific job—and when you consume too much sugar, it's like sending a disruptive force into this community.

Excessive sugar can upset the balance of good and bad bacteria in your gut and lead to a condition known as dysbiosis, where the harmony within your gut community is disturbed. Why does this matter for mental health? Well, the gut and the brain have a constant line of communication, often referred to as the gut-brain axis.

When the gut microbiome is out of balance, it can send signals to the brain that might influence mood and emotions. Some studies even suggest that an unhealthy gut microbiome could be linked to mental health issues, including feelings of anxiety and depression (Clapp et al., 2017). If you're interested in exploring the fascinating link between gut health and brain function further, you can read another one of my books, part of this Brain Health & Wellbeing series, which delves into the connections of the gut-brain relationship. Please see the Appendix to be updated on relevant books in this series.

Ultra-processed foods (UPFs) often contain emulsifiers and preservatives that can disrupt your gut microbiome. Additionally, the ultra-processing method and hidden sugars in UPFs can cause blood sugar spikes. UPFs are designed to be highly palatable which often leads to overconsumption. If you are interested to learn more, please check out my book: *Quit Ultra-Processed Foods Now*, where I share a practical 6-step strategy to transition away from UPFs, via this link: **https://books2read.com/quitupf**

Key Takeaways

This chapter highlighted the connection between what we eat and how it affects our mood and mental well-being.

- Fluctuations in blood glucose levels impact emotional stability and are also associated with serious mood disorders such as anxiety and bipolar disorder. The brain and endocrine system collaborate to control mood, with neurotransmitters such as serotonin and dopamine affected by fluctuations in blood sugar.

- Insulin, released in response to glucose, helps cells absorb glucose for energy. Imbalances in blood glucose can disrupt insulin function and affect how cells use glucose. Hormones like cortisol, related to stress, are also influenced by blood glucose fluctuations, impacting emotional responses.

- Balanced dietary choices and lifestyle measures such as sleep, physical activity, mindfulness and stress management, can support stable blood glucose levels.

***

The next chapter will enlighten us on the long-term effects of dysregulated blood glucose on brain health.

Theme 2:

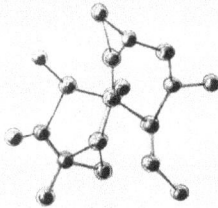

When Things Go Wrong

Chapter 5:

The Long-Term Effects of Dysregulated Blood Glucose on Brain Health

Do you know how long-term dysregulated blood glucose could affect your brain health? Digging deeper into this question uncovers a complicated relationship between blood sugar changes and different aspects of brain function and structure.

Chronic Hyperglycemia and Cognitive Decline

While brief spikes in blood glucose can momentarily impact cognitive function, the real concern lies in chronic hyperglycemia, or the sustained elevation of blood sugar levels over time. This prolonged exposure has profound and enduring consequences for brain health, increasing the risk of cognitive decline and neurodegenerative conditions.

Persistently elevated glucose levels contribute to the formation of advanced glycation end-products (AGEs). These compounds can accumulate in various tissues, including the brain, and have been associated with inflammation and oxidative stress, both of which are issues for neuronal health (Twarda-Clapa et al., 2022). This persistent inflammation may impair concentration and memory and increase the risk of severe conditions such as dementia.

Chronic elevation of blood glucose levels can lead to increased oxidative stress, as well. This imbalance between antioxidants and free radicals may damage mitochondria and cells, including neurons, and contribute to the aging of the brain. Chronic hyperglycemia is also closely linked to insulin resistance, where cells become less responsive to insulin. Since insulin plays a crucial role in brain function, its impairment can negatively impact cognitive processes.

Additionally, prolonged exposure to elevated glucose levels may contribute to the dysfunction of the blood-brain barrier, a protective barrier that regulates the passage of substances into the brain. This can potentially allow harmful substances to enter the brain, impacting its health. The balance of neurotransmitters can be influenced by elevated glucose levels as well, affecting communication between neurons. This disruption in signaling may contribute to cognitive impairments.

Insulin Resistance and Its Impact on the Brain

When insulin resistance occurs, glucose faces obstacles in entering our brain cells, leading to reduced availability of this vital energy source. Impaired glucose uptake can result in energy deficits. The consequences of this can manifest as cognitive dysfunction. This may include difficulties in concentration, memory lapses, and an overall decline in cognitive performance.

In addition to glucose management, insulin also serves as a shield for brain cells, preserving their well-being and supporting optimal cognitive function. However, when insulin resistance occurs, this dismantles the neuroprotective role provided by insulin. This can leave brain cells vulnerable to various stressors and potential damage. The consequences of this can be far-reaching. Cognitive decline becomes a concern as the brain's defense mechanisms are weakened.

Insulin Resistance and Alzheimer's Disease

Recognizing the strong association between insulin resistance and Alzheimer's disease has led to Alzheimer's disease being referred to as "type 3 diabetes" by some scientists (de la Monte & Wands, 2008).

Just as diabetes affects the body's ability to manage blood sugar, insulin resistance, which is a key aspect of type 2 diabetes, impacts more than just glucose control. It sets off a series of events that contribute to the development and progression of Alzheimer's disease. This highlights the importance of maintaining insulin sensitivity for overall brain health.

Understanding Alzheimer's disease as "type 3 diabetes" in some people emphasizes that this neurodegenerative condition is not only about memory loss but also involves connections with metabolic processes, particularly those regulated by insulin.

Vascular Health, Blood Glucose, and the Brain

When we talk about poor blood glucose control, we're referring to difficulties in managing the sugar levels in our bloodstream. Imagine your blood vessels as delicate highways that need to stay clear and functional for everything to run smoothly. In cases where blood glucose is consistently high, it can cause damage to these vital transportation networks, our blood vessels. It's like a constant high tide eroding the edges of a riverbank. This continuous stress on the vessels can lead to a condition known as vascular dementia.

Vascular dementia occurs when the brain doesn't receive enough blood and, hence, not enough oxygen and nutrients. Picture them as interruptions in the smooth flow of traffic along those highways. These interruptions, caused by the impaired blood vessels, can affect our cognitive functions.

There are a couple of mechanisms by which poor glucose control can lead to damage to the blood vessels:

- The inner lining of blood vessels, called the endothelium, can be impaired by high sugar levels. This dysfunction reduces the ability of blood vessels to regulate blood flow and maintain balance in the body.

- High blood sugar triggers an inflammatory response in the body. This inflammation can damage the blood vessel walls, making them more susceptible to various issues.

- Excess sugar in the bloodstream can lead to the formation of AGEs. These compounds can accumulate in blood vessels, promoting stiffness and reducing their flexibility.

- Elevated glucose levels contribute to increased oxidative stress, where there's an imbalance between the production of free radicals and the body's ability to counteract them. This oxidative stress can harm blood vessel tissues.

- High blood sugar can lead to an increase in the thickness of the blood. This makes it harder for blood to flow smoothly through the vessels, putting additional strain on them.

Impact of Glycemic Variability on Cerebral Blood Flow

Remember our earlier discussion about glycemic variability? Well, it's time to connect the dots and understand how those fluctuations in blood glucose levels can play a role in cerebral blood flow, influencing our brain health and function.

Glycemic variability refers to the fluctuations in blood sugar levels over time. These ups and downs can have a notable impact on the blood vessels, including those that supply blood to the brain. Here's how it unfolds:

Sudden spikes and drops in blood glucose levels trigger a response in the blood vessels. Rapid increases may lead to a dilation (widening) of blood vessels, while sharp decreases can cause constriction (narrowing). Over time, these dynamic changes affect overall cerebral blood flow (Corinne O'Keefe Osborn, 2017).

The brain is a highly sensitive organ that requires a consistent and well-regulated blood supply to function optimally. Glycemic variability can disrupt this balance. When blood flow to the brain fluctuates, it can impact cognitive functions such as memory, attention, and overall mental sharpness.

Prolonged glycemic variability is associated with microvascular damage, affecting the smaller blood vessels. This damage can compromise the integrity of the blood-brain barrier, a protective barrier that regulates the passage of substances between the bloodstream and the brain.

Fluctuations in blood sugar levels also contribute to an inflammatory response in the body. This inflammation can extend to the blood vessels, further affecting cerebral blood flow and potentially contributing to long-term damage.

Preventive Strategies for Vascular Health

Luckily, there are some practical lifestyle and dietary tips that you can easily incorporate into your daily routine to protect the health of your blood vessels:

- **Balanced diet:** Aim for a balanced and varied diet rich in fruits, vegetables, whole grains, lean proteins, and healthy fats. This provides essential nutrients that support overall vascular health.

- **Hydration:** Stay well-hydrated by drinking an adequate amount of water throughout the day. Proper hydration supports circulation and helps maintain the flexibility of blood vessels.

- **Regular physical activity:** Engage in regular physical activity, such as walking, jogging, or other forms of exercise. Physical exercise promotes healthy blood circulation and contributes to vascular flexibility.

- **Avoid smoking:** If you smoke, consider quitting or cutting down on the amount. Smoking is a major risk factor for vascular damage, and quitting can significantly improve vascular health.

- **Manage stress:** Practice stress-reducing techniques like deep breathing, meditation, or yoga. Chronic stress can contribute to vascular issues, and managing stress positively impacts overall well-being.

- **Limit ultra-processed foods:** Reduce your intake of ultra-processed and sugary foods. Opt for whole, nutrient-dense foods to provide your body with necessary nutrients without unnecessary additives.

- **Control blood pressure and cholesterol:** Regularly monitor and manage blood pressure and cholesterol levels. High blood pressure and elevated cholesterol can strain your blood vessels.

- **Adequate sleep:** Ensure you get sufficient, quality sleep. Sleep is crucial for overall health, including vascular and brain health.

- **Moderate alcohol consumption:** If you consume alcohol, do so in moderation. Excessive alcohol intake can contribute to vascular and brain health issues, so it's important to limit your intake.

- **Regular health check-ups:** Schedule regular visits to your healthcare provider to monitor key health indicators and catch any potential issues early.

Preventing Brain Atrophy with Blood Glucose Control

As we age, our brains naturally undergo a process of shrinkage known as brain atrophy. This can be accelerated by poor blood glucose control, leading to the gradual loss or shrinking of brain cells and tissues. Chronic health conditions or diseases can exacerbate this process, impacting cognitive functions and increasing the risk of neurological issues.

Managing blood glucose levels plays a crucial role in preventing or slowing brain atrophy by ensuring a consistent and balanced energy supply to support brain cell functions. Fluctuations in blood glucose, especially elevated levels, contribute to oxidative stress, damaging brain cells over time. Additionally, elevated blood glucose levels can impact blood vessel health, disrupting proper blood flow to the brain and affecting neurotransmitter function, which is essential for efficient communication between brain cells and cognitive health.

Research indicates a significant connection between blood glucose management and brain volume. Consistently high levels may lead to a decline in brain volume, particularly in regions critical for memory and decision-making. On the contrary, well-managed blood glucose levels are associated with better preservation of brain volume, potentially mitigating age-related cognitive decline (Edwards, 2016).

Impact of Blood Glucose on Mitochondrial Health in the Brain

In an earlier chapter we covered how the mitochondria are vital cellular components responsible for generating energy. High or low blood glucose levels can disrupt this energy production process, leading to what we call mitochondrial dysfunction. It's like a fluctuating power source affecting the functioning of electronic devices. In the brain, this dysfunction can lead to problems—like damage to the neurons, the building blocks of our brain.

In conditions where blood glucose levels are consistently high, such as in diabetes, mitochondria may face oxidative stress and inflammation, affecting their ability to produce energy efficiently. On the other hand, low glucose levels can deprive mitochondria of the necessary fuel for energy production, also compromising their function. As a result, impaired mitochondrial function can disrupt the energy supply to neurons, leading to potential damage and dysfunction.

Therapeutic Approaches Targeting Mitochondria

Therapeutic approaches and lifestyle interventions with a focus on improving mitochondrial function may counteract the effects of blood glucose imbalances on brain health. These strategies aim to support the optimal performance of mitochondria, which is crucial for the energy needs of brain cells. Here are some avenues worth exploring:

- **Regular exercise:** Engaging in regular exercise has been associated with improved mitochondrial function. Physical activity promotes mitochondrial biogenesis, the process of creating new mitochondria, and enhances their efficiency in producing energy.

- **Balanced diet:** Adopting a balanced and nutrient-rich diet can positively impact mitochondrial health. Including foods rich in antioxidants and essential nutrients and maintaining an appropriate calorie balance supports mitochondrial function.

- **Fasting:** Periods of fasting, when done safely and under guidance, have been linked to enhanced mitochondrial function. This practice may stimulate cellular processes, including autophagy, which can contribute to mitochondrial renewal.

- **Supplements:** Some supplements are designed to specifically support mitochondrial function. Coenzyme Q10 (CoQ10) and alpha-lipoic acid are examples of antioxidants that may benefit mitochondrial health (National Institutes of Health, n.d.).

- **Stress management:** Chronic stress can contribute to mitochondrial dysfunction. Implementing stress-management techniques, such as mindfulness and relaxation exercises, may positively influence mitochondrial health.

- **Quality sleep:** This is essential for overall health, including mitochondrial function. Establishing good sleep hygiene practices can contribute to the restoration and efficiency of mitochondria.

You may be glad to know that the above strategies for improving your mitochondrial health also has a positive effect on blood sugar regulation and your brain health! We delve deeper into these lifestyle factors and interventions, in the next section of this book.

Key Takeaways

In this chapter, we've explored the enduring consequences of blood glucose on brain health. Here are a few key takeaways that will empower you with the knowledge to navigate the relationship between blood glucose and the sustained health of your brain.

- Your daily lifestyle choices, such as exercise, nutrition, and stress management, play a pivotal role in supporting both blood glucose control and the health of your brain.

- Chronic imbalances in blood glucose can accelerate brain aging and increase your risk of neurodegenerative diseases. Prioritizing stable levels is a proactive approach to long-term cognitive health.

- Explore lifestyle interventions and therapeutic strategies to boost mitochondrial function, offering potential protection against the adverse effects of blood glucose imbalances.

- Every individual is unique. Tailor your approach to blood glucose control and brain health based on your specific needs, and consult healthcare professionals for personalized guidance.

***

In Chapter 6, we'll delve into the impact of your diet on the health of your brain.

Theme 3:

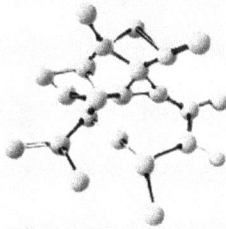

Practical Strategies for Blood Sugar Regulation to Enhance Brain Health

Chapter 6:
Diet and Its Impact on Brain Energy

When you're feeling low in energy, grabbing a quick sugary snack for a boost might seem like a good idea, but the brain's reaction may be more like a roller coaster than a steady climb.

These choices don't just affect your immediate focus; they may leave a longer-lasting impact on your brain. Think of your choices like planting seeds—the meals you choose today can influence how your brain functions in the long run.

Understanding the Glycemic Index

The glycemic index (GI) is your guide in the world of food, helping you to find the right balance for your mental health. This tool reveals how quickly different foods can affect our blood sugar.

Choosing a diet rich in low-GI foods, such as certain types of fruits and vegetables, lays the foundation for stable blood sugar levels. These foods release glucose gradually, avoiding sudden spikes and crashes and providing a consistent and reliable fuel supply for the body and brain.

Conversely, high-GI foods can initiate a rollercoaster ride for blood sugar levels. When you consume high-GI foods, such as sugary snacks or refined grains like white bread, the body digests them quickly, causing blood sugar levels to spike.

This rapid increase in blood sugar triggers the pancreas to release insulin in an attempt to regulate glucose levels. You may recall that in Chapter 3, we covered how a surge in insulin in response to a blood sugar spike can sometimes lead to an overcorrection, causing blood sugar levels to drop rapidly.

This leads to a crash in energy levels—a phenomenon commonly referred to as the "sugar crash." This cycle of rapid spikes and subsequent crashes in blood sugar levels can contribute to feelings of fatigue, hunger, and irritability, ultimately affecting overall energy levels and cognitive function.

In essence, our dietary decisions play a crucial role in the stability of our blood sugar levels, influencing mood and mental health. Opting for a low-GI diet creates a supportive environment for the mind, fostering emotional balance and overall well-being.

Low-GI Foods

Foods with low GI ratings gradually release glucose into the blood stream. Think of foods with a GI rating of 55 or below as a gentle stream, providing a sustained and steady energy flow (Ajimera, 2020).

Medium-GI Foods

With moderate GI ratings (56–69), these foods release glucose at a moderate pace (Ajimera, 2020). Picture it as a flowing river—not too slow, not too fast—ensuring a balanced and manageable increase in blood sugar levels.

High-GI Foods

Foods with high GI ratings (70 or above) cause a rapid surge in blood sugar levels.

Understanding these GI ratings empowers us to make choices aligned with our health goals. Balancing our diet with a mix of low- and medium-

GI foods supports stable blood sugar levels, contributing to overall well-being.

Here is a table categorizing some of the common foods we tend to consume, listed here according to their GI ratings:

Glycemic Index	Examples of Foods
Low-GI (0-55)	Soy products (tofu, tempeh), beans (chickpeas, kidney beans, pinto beans, black beans, and navy beans), grapefruit, apricots, apples, watermelons, milk, and porridge (oats)
Medium-GI (56-69)	Orange juice, honey, basmati rice, and wholemeal bread
High-GI (70 or above)	Potatoes, white bread, and short-grain rice.

This table here is a guide, created using a helpful resource from The University of Sydney: glycemicindex.com/gi-search/

Please note that individual responses may vary, influenced by other factors such as sleep, gut health, and stress levels. So, we suggest that you use the above table or weblink as a guide only to plan your meals and snacks, and tailor this by observing your own energy levels 30-120 minutes after eating.

Glycemic Load and Brain Function

Now let's look at the Glycemic Load (GL). Think of GL as the upgraded version of GI to balance your blood sugar levels.

While the GI focuses on individual foods, the GL takes into account both the quality and quantity of carbohydrates, as well as the impact of eating carbohydrates in combination with other macronutrients (e.g. fats and protein).

This gives us a more comprehensive view of how a particular food affects our blood sugar. This knowledge is helpful because we can combine foods in meals in a way that allows us to enjoy food with a higher GI while minimizing spikes in our blood sugar levels.

A diet with a low glycemic load provides a steady and sustained supply of glucose to the brain. This helps avoid the energy fluctuations of high and low blood sugar, supports stable cognitive function, and maintains consistent energy levels throughout the day.

Balancing Macronutrients for Optimal Brain Energy

Let's explore some nutrition tips in the context of low-GI/GL foods and additional ways to stabilize blood sugar for your brain health.

You know how your car needs the right fuel to run smoothly? Well, think of your brain the same way. It's this incredible powerhouse that craves a blend of nutrients to keep it firing on all cylinders.

A well-balanced diet is integral to maintaining stable blood glucose levels and supporting optimal brain health. Key components of such a diet include whole grains, lean proteins, healthy fats, fruits, and vegetables.

Carbohydrates for Sustained Energy

Eating carbohydrates from low-to-medium GI/GL sources like whole grains, e.g. brown rice and whole-wheat bread, are valuable sources of sustained energy. These grains are rich in complex carbohydrates and fiber, which take longer to digest, providing a steady release of glucose into the bloodstream. This sustained energy release helps maintain stable blood glucose levels, supporting the brain's continuous need for fuel.

Fiber

In addition to fiber from whole grains, this can also be consumed from fruits and vegetables, which are abundant in antioxidants and essential vitamins for a healthy metabolism. Antioxidants help neutralize harmful free radicals, protecting the brain and mitochondria from oxidative stress and inflammation. We covered the importance of antioxidant defense in Chapter 2 on mitochondria and brain energy metabolism.

Additionally, vitamins in plant-based foods such as vitamin C, vitamin E, and folate play key roles in cognitive function and overall brain health. Phytonutrients which give the plants their color are powerful antioxidants and supports gut health. We will cover more about gut health and glucose in Chapter 8.

It is best to consume fruits in moderation due to the amount of sugar in them. You may wish to check out the GI of your favorite fruit using this resource from The University of Sydney: glycemicindex.com/gi-search/. Fruit juices tend to cause a sharp rise in blood sugar because most of the fruit's fiber is removed during processing. If you consume fruit smoothies, consider adding nut butters, avocado and vegetables to reduce their GL.

Healthy Fats and Cognitive Health

Fats help keep the brain's machinery running smoothly, like oil in a machine. Fatty acids which come from the breakdown of fats we eat, are essential components of the membranes in our brain cells. They contribute to the structure and function of neurons, the cells responsible for transmitting information in the brain.

Healthy fats, found in foods such as avocados, nuts, fatty fish, and olive oil, support good brain health. These fats, particularly omega-3 fatty acids, contribute to the formation of cell membranes and assist in maintaining the flexibility and integrity of these membranes, ensuring the smooth operation of various cognitive functions.

Omega-3 fatty acids, found in foods like fatty fish (salmon, mackerel, and sardines), flaxseed, and walnuts, are particularly vital. They have anti-inflammatory properties, helping to maintain a healthy environment in the brain (Zivkovic et al., 2011). DHA (docosahexaenoic acid), a type of omega-3, is a major structural component of brain cell membranes.

Although plant-based omega-3 sources (like flaxseeds, chia seeds, and walnuts) offer fiber and phytonutrients, the body's limited ability to process these compounds means we get less omega-3 from them. Therefore, considering marine-based sources can be helpful. This could mean eating fatty fish at least twice a week or taking omega-3 supplements derived from fish or algae. When selecting omega-3 supplements, look for those tested by third parties or with Good Manufacturing Practice certification. This ensures the supplements are free from contaminants like heavy metals and contain the stated amount of omega-3.

Omega-6 fatty acids, present in nuts, seeds and vegetable oils, are also necessary for various physiological processes. However excessive consumption e.g. with ultra-processed foods or food fried in high amounts of vegetable oils, may lead to inflammation.

A balance between omega-3 and omega-6 is crucial for optimal brain function. Both types of fatty acids contribute to the complex network of signals in the brain, influencing cognitive processes, neurotransmitter function, and overall brain health. Including a variety of sources of these fatty acids in your diet helps provide the building blocks necessary for maintaining a healthy and well-functioning brain.

There are also omega-9 fatty acids, found in abundance in foods such as olive oil and avocados. These play a vital role in promoting and maintaining brain health. While they are not classified as essential fatty acids, their contribution to supporting the structure and function of brain cells is considerable. These fatty acids facilitate the smooth functioning of individual brain cells, promote cell integrity, ensure efficient communication between neurons, and contribute to the overall resilience and vitality of the brain.

Proteins for the Brain and Satiety

Dietary proteins play a fundamental role in the synthesis of neurotransmitters, for communication within the brain and critical for various cognitive processes. When you consume protein-rich foods like beans, lentils, meat, fish, and nuts, your body breaks down these proteins into amino acids, the building blocks essential for neurotransmitter synthesis.

These neurotransmitters facilitate communication between different brain regions, regulating mood, memory formation, and cognitive function. By supporting neurotransmitter production, amino acids derived from protein-rich foods promote efficient brain communication, enhancing various cognitive processes like emotion regulation, memory retention, and information processing, thus contributing to optimal brain health and performance.

Proteins act as the brain's building blocks, helping repair and grow things in the brain. Additionally, proteins play an important role in promoting the feeling of fullness after eating, curbing cravings and preventing unnecessary snacking.

This phenomenon may be related to the protein leverage hypothesis, which proposes that the body regulates food intake based on the consumption of protein-rich foods, prioritizing their consumption to meet nutritional needs and maintain a sense of fullness. Thus, incorporating adequate protein into our diet not only supports brain health but also aids in managing appetite and promoting overall well-being.

Lean proteins can be derived from foods like beans, lentils, nuts, and fish. Protein sourced from beans and lentils also provide the additional benefits of phytonutrients and fiber, highlighted previously.

Personalizing Your Healthy Eating Plate

I often get asked about the optimal ratio of proteins, fats and carbohydrates. There are various views on this, and I take the approach of personalizing this to the individual. For example, an athlete would need more carbohydrates to fuel their physical training, and an office worker may need less of it. The optimal ratio may also need to be adjusted according to any pre-existing health conditions or medications, so please discuss this first with your healthcare practitioner.

I usually suggest people start by observing what they are currently doing, how this impacts their health and energy levels, and tailor this accordingly. A good starting benchmark for a Healthy Eating Plate is 40-50% non-starchy vegetables, approximately 25% lean protein, 25% carbohydrates from whole grains or root vegetables, and a small amount of healthy fats, for example from avocado, seeds and nuts. Eating healthy fats with your meals also slow down digestion, preventing rapid spikes in blood sugar and promoting sustained energy.

You can see a visual example of a Healthy Eating Plate, on the Harvard T.H. Chan School of Public Health webpage: **https://nutritionsource.hsph.harvard.edu/healthy-eating-plate/**

For people who have not been consuming vegetables regularly, I recommend they gradually increase the amount of vegetable intake, to help their digestive tract adjust to the increasing fiber intake. Aim for a variety of non-starchy vegetables, up to 5 servings or more daily. You may find it helpful to use this free resource created by Dr Michael Greger that helps people track their daily intake of fruit and fiber, see **https://nutritionfacts.org/daily-dozen/**

More Nutrition Tips for Stabilizing Your Blood Sugar

Impact of Meal Patterns on Brain Energy

Breakfast is often hailed as the most important meal of the day, and for good reason. Starting your day with the right meal that helps stabilize blood sugar levels can significantly enhance your concentration and cognitive performance. A well-balanced high protein breakfast also lays the groundwork for maintaining optimal blood sugar control throughout the day, thereby fostering sustained mental focus and overall well-being.

Whether you consume breakfast or not, make note of your energy levels to help you decide what your body needs. Again, discuss this with your healthcare practitioner if you have a co-existing condition or on medication.

In addition to breakfast, the timing and frequency of your meals will shape the availability of energy for your brain throughout the day. The human body follows a circadian rhythm, a natural cycle that controls the sleep-wake pattern and repeats approximately every 24 hours. This rhythm affects many biological functions, including metabolism—your body's internal clock helps determine how effectively it digests food and utilizes energy.

For example, a research study found that carbohydrate-rich meals are processed more effectively when eaten earlier in the day, especially in people with impaired glucose regulation (Kessler et al, 2017). Based on these findings, the researchers recommended that people with impaired glucose metabolism avoid large, carbohydrate-rich dinners.

Regular and balanced meals spaced throughout the day contribute to a more consistent supply of nutrients, including glucose. Erratic eating habits may impact blood sugar levels and your brain's ability to maintain steady energy. Such fluctuations can result in feelings of fatigue, irritability, and difficulty concentrating.

Mindful Snacking

Consider if well-timed snacks can be helpful for you. For example, if you notice an energy dip or hunger pang mid-afternoon, when you would usually grab a chocolate bar or snack from the vending machine, it may be helpful to look at your lunchtime meal composition. If this is already optimized for blood sugar balance with the above strategies, you may wish to consider a well-timed snack just before this energy dip. Opt for snacks with a combination of protein and fiber to keep you satiated between meals. Examples include veggies with hummus, handful of nuts with an apple, or roasted chocolate chickpeas. If you would like a free copy of my roasted chickpea recipe, please see the Appendix for details!

Choose Vegetables First

Starting your meal with the non-starchy vegetables slows down the absorption of carbohydrates. For example, eat the non-starchy vegetables on your dinner plate first before the starchy carbohydrates. The fiber in these non-starchy vegetables slows down the absorption of carbohydrates. This help regulate blood sugar levels and reduce glycemic fluctuations.

If you have a starter before your main meal, consider a leafy salad or vegetable soup. This can help stabilize your blood sugar response to carbohydrates consumed during the rest of your meal.

Save Desserts for Last

Eating your dessert after a main meal can help limit blood sugar spikes. This allows for a gentler increase in blood sugar, as the main meal slows down digestion. However, it's still important to watch your portion size to minimize the impact on blood sugar levels.

Portion Sizes

Be mindful of portion sizes to avoid overeating. Smaller, well-balanced meals with a low GL spread throughout the day can prevent rapid spikes and drops in blood sugar. This is especially important for those managing diabetes or aiming to regulate glycemic variability.

Make Resistant Starch

Another method to consider is adding resistant starch to your diet, which is formed by cooking and rapidly cooling starchy foods such as rice, pasta or potatoes. Resistant starch does not get absorbed by the body but passes into the large intestine where it feeds the gut bacteria and can benefit gut health.

To decrease the glycemic index of starches, try cooking them, and letting them cool rapidly. I also likely a add a splash of extra-virgin olive oil as the starches cool. If you wish to eat your meals hot, you can reheat them before eating. This approach reduces the chance of sudden blood sugar spikes.

Reduce your AGE

You may recall that in the last chapter that stabilizing blood glucose can prevent the formation of advanced glycation end-products (AGEs). The damaging effect of AGEs include inflammation and oxidative stress, leading to stiffening of blood vessel walls and reduced blood flow to brain cells.

Cooking methods are another consideration, as this can reduce dietary AGE intake by up to 50% (Uribarri et al., 2010). Animal-derived foods high in fat and protein are prone to AGE formation during cooking with high-heat methods like frying, grilling, roasting. Instead, opt for steaming, boiling or slow cooking. Marinating food in lemon juice or vinegar before cooking can also reduce AGE formation.

Foods such as vegetables, fruits and whole grains contain relatively few AGEs, even after cooking (Uribarri et al., 2010).

Flaxseed and Blueberries

Flaxseeds and blueberries are two versatile superfoods that can help stabilize blood sugar response (Morreira et al., 2022; Stull, 2016). Consider adding them to various meals throughout your day. For example, sprinkle them on top of your breakfast porridge, add them to desserts, and include them when baking. I also like to sprinkle cinnamon on top (more about this in Chapter 8)!

Vinegar

Having vinegar with meals can improve blood sugar response and insulin sensitivity (Shishehbor et al., 2017). Consider adding a vinaigrette made of vinegar and cold-pressed, extra-virgin olive oil to your meals. For example, sprinkled over salads, or use it for dipping bread.

Limit Ultra-Processed Foods

One category of foods to be cautious about is ultra-processed foods (UPFs).

UPFs often contain sugar, which can be hidden and not immediately obvious unless you scrutinize the labels. These foods are designed to be highly palatable, leading to overeating.

Reduce your intake of UPFs, as they often have higher GI values. Instead, focus on whole, minimally processed options to support stable blood sugar.

UPFs often contain added ingredients such as emulsifiers and preservatives which can affect gut health, and the gut-brain axis. For a more in-depth exploration of this, please check out my book *Quit Ultra-Processed Foods Now*, which delves into the effects of such additives on the gut microbiome and overall well-being. In this book I also share a practical 6-step strategy to transition away from UPFs. More details about the book in the Appendix, and via this link: **https://books2read.com/quitupf**

Pre-Plan your Shopping Trip

Pre-plan your grocery shopping trip to stock up on whole foods with low-to-moderate GI, and ingredients to create low-to-moderate GL meals. This can help avoid impulsive purchases, particularly when you're tired or hungry. Also, stock up on organic seeds and nuts. These are versatile ingredients that reduce GL, while adding healthy fats, fiber, and phytonutrients to your meals.

Additional Considerations

Ketogenic Diet and Brain Metabolism

As shared in Chapter 2, there may be situations where a ketogenic diet can be a therapeutic strategy. It's beyond the scope of this book to cover ketogenic diet in detail, so I encourage you to research high-quality and reputable resources if you're considering this approach. If so, it's important to pursue it in a healthy manner. Be cautious about unhealthy practices, such as relying solely on meat or processed foods. For safe and effective implementation, consult a healthcare practitioner or certified nutritionist to ensure it aligns with your individual health needs.

Hydration for Your Brain and Blood Sugar

How often do you consider water to be a fundamental part of a healthy diet? Water is not just a thirst quencher; it's a key player in supporting various bodily functions, including those critical to the brain. Dehydration, even in mild forms, can have noticeable impacts on cognitive abilities. From difficulty concentrating to increased feelings of fatigue, the consequences of inadequate hydration extend beyond mere thirst.

Recent studies have found a connection between not drinking enough water and difficulties managing blood sugar levels, especially in people with Type 2 Diabetes. This means that when your body doesn't have enough water, it might struggle to keep your blood sugar at the right level (Zaplatosch & Adams, 2020).

The reason behind this is a hormone called arginine vasopressin (AVP), which helps control how much water your body holds onto. When you're low on water, your body releases more AVP to hold on to whatever water it has. However, this can impact how your body handles sugar. It's important to stay hydrated to help your body better manage your blood sugar.

How does that thirsty feeling hit you? It's unpleasant, isn't it? By the time you sense that thirst, however, your brain has already felt the impact double-fold.

When you're not drinking enough water, trying to focus feels like trying to navigate through a fog. It gets tough, and your attention slips away easily.

Dehydration can also make your memory a bit tricky, and you'll find yourself searching for details that would easily come to you when you're well hydrated.

Think of water as the delivery person who brings packages to your doorstep. Water moves essential nutrients to your brain. These nutrients include the ones you get from foods, like vitamins and minerals, as well as glucose, the brain's main energy source.

When you eat, your body breaks down the food into these valuable nutrients. Water acts as the carrier, transporting them through your bloodstream and making sure your brain gets the fuel it needs to function at its best.

After your brain has used up the nutrients delivered by water, there are by-products and waste that need to be removed to keep things clean and healthy. Water acts as the cleanup crew, flushing out these waste products and toxins that could potentially cause harm. This cleansing process is vital for maintaining a pristine environment within your brain.

General guidelines recommend about 8 glasses (64 ounces) of water per day, but individual needs vary based on factors like age, weight, activity level, and climate. It's essential to listen to your body's signals of thirst and aim to drink water regularly throughout the day to maintain proper hydration levels and support brain health.

Electrolytes helps with hydration balance at a cellular level. Think of them as tiny messengers in your body. Among these messengers, sodium functions as a regulator of fluid balance within and around cells. Its role can be likened to that of a traffic controller, ensuring a balanced flow of water into and out of cells, thereby significantly contributing to the maintenance of hydration levels.

Potassium operates as a stabilizing force. By balancing the effects of sodium, potassium prevents cellular overload with water. This harmonious relationship is fundamental to creating an environment conducive to effective communication among brain cells.

Magnesium, the third essential electrolyte, assumes the role of a versatile facilitator. It is instrumental in numerous biochemical processes, particularly those vital to brain function. Its impact extends to supporting neurotransmitter function, thereby enhancing the smooth transmission of signals within the neural network.

While staying adequately hydrated is crucial for optimal brain function, it's equally important to be aware of the potential risks associated with excessive water intake. Hyponatremia, a condition arising from dangerously diluted sodium levels in the body, poses a significant danger.

The repercussions can range from mild confusion to severe seizures, and in extreme cases, it may even result in a coma.

To avoid such risks, approach hydration with moderation. Maintain a balanced flow in the hydration dance—not so little to cause dehydration but also not too much to wash out the crucial electrolytes like sodium, potassium, and magnesium. Striking this balance ensures your brain functions optimally, benefiting from both the virtues of hydration and the stability of electrolyte levels. A general rule of thumb is that when one is adequately hydrated the urine is slightly straw colored.

Your body will naturally derive electrolytes from eating a variety of fruits and vegetables. On hot days, consider snacking on more vegetables, eat fruits such as watermelon, or drink coconut water. If possible, avoid sugary drinks or fruit juices that may spike your blood sugar levels.

High-Mercury Fish

If you are considering fish as your protein source, note that high-mercury fish pose a specific concern when it comes to brain health. Certain types of fish, such as shark, swordfish, king mackerel, and tilefish, are known to contain elevated levels of mercury. Mercury is a neurotoxin, meaning it can be harmful to the nervous system, and it poses particular risks to brain health.

When we consume fish with a high mercury content, this neurotoxin can accumulate in our bodies over time. This accumulation may lead to adverse effects on brain function and is of particular concern during critical periods of development, such as pregnancy. Exposure to mercury during pregnancy can harm the developing fetal brain and nervous system, potentially leading to cognitive and developmental issues in the child.

Glucose Checks and Medication Review

Before you start adjusting your diet, please first discuss with your healthcare professional if you have a pre-existing condition or on medications. This is particularly important to people taking medication for diabetes as you may require more regular blood glucose checks and medication review, as you embark on new dietary strategies.

Key Takeaways

This chapter has explored the impact of diet on our brain health. Here are a few key points to consider:

- Erratic meals or consuming the wrong foods can disrupt cognitive function.

- Sugary snacks may provide a quick boost, but they cause fluctuations in blood sugar that can affect the brain.

- By incorporating low- and medium- GI foods into your diet and following practical tips like seeking the GI symbol, embracing non-starchy vegetables, and mindful snacking, you can effectively manage your blood sugar levels, supporting stable energy and cognitive function throughout the day.

- Whole grains offer sustained energy, lean proteins support cognitive sharpness, healthy fats (omega-3) are vital for brain cell structure, and fruits and vegetables provide antioxidants.

- Water is a fundamental part of brain metabolism, acting as a delivery system for nutrients and a cleanser of waste products.

- Thirst is a late indicator of dehydration, with cognitive impacts already underway.

- Hydration is not just important for optimal brain function, it also helps balance blood sugar levels

***

The coming chapter will equip you with more lifestyle strategies to balance your blood sugar levels for your brain health.

Chapter 7:
Lifestyle Choices for Optimal Brain Function

Have you ever had a day when your body and mind felt drained, like they needed a reset button? We've all been there, and in the moment, it feels like there isn't much you can do to exit this funk. Fortunately, by boosting your brain function, you can rejuvenate both your body and mind, leaving you feeling refreshed and ready to take on the world.

Keep in mind that every aspect of your routine, from getting enough sleep to staying active, significantly influences how your brain performs. To unlock its full potential, consider these effective adjustments you can make to your lifestyle.

Exercise and Physical Activity for Brain and Glucose Benefits

Exercise and physical activity not only impacts our physical health but also plays a significant role in regulating blood glucose levels and supporting brain function. When you engage in physical activity, your muscles actively take up glucose from the bloodstream, helping to stabilize blood sugar levels. This improves insulin sensitivity and stabilizes blood sugar levels. This process is crucial for maintaining overall metabolic balance and preventing fluctuations in glucose levels that can negatively affect brain function.

Through exercise, your brain also becomes more skilled at absorbing and utilizing glucose, leading to enhanced cognitive functions such as improved memory, focus, and problem-solving abilities.

Types of Exercise and Their Effects on Brain and Blood Glucose

Various forms of exercise bring about different impacts on your body, and equally, they influence your brain glucose levels in distinct ways. Understanding these differences can help you tailor your exercise routine to optimize its benefits for your cognitive health.

- **Aerobic Exercise:** Aerobic exercises, which increase heart rate and breathing, have profound benefits for the brain. Activities like brisk walking, running, swimming, and cycling fall into this category. Aerobic exercise enhances blood flow, delivering essential nutrients and oxygen to the brain. It also promotes the release of neurotransmitters like dopamine and serotonin, contributing to improved mood and cognitive function.

  Moreover, aerobic exercise is particularly beneficial for training metabolic flexibility, allowing the body to efficiently use fatty acids as an alternative energy source (Attia & Gifford, 2023). This adaptation enhances the brain's ability to maintain optimal function, even during periods of fluctuating glucose availability.

- **Strength Training:** Strength training, involving resistance exercises to build muscle strength, is not only beneficial for the body but also for brain health. Weightlifting, resistance band exercises, and bodyweight workouts like push-ups and squats are examples. Strength training enhances neural connections and releases growth factors in the brain, which repair and maintain brain cells.

  With regular strength training, you can build and maintain muscle, which is an important organ for metabolic health and blood glucose regulation.

- **High-Intensity Interval Training (HIIT):** HIIT combines short bursts of intense activity with brief rest periods. It has been shown to enhance glucose metabolism in the brain, contributing to improved cognitive performance (Robinson et al., 2018).

- **Flexibility Exercises:** Flexibility exercises, including stretching and yoga, contribute to overall brain health and improve balance, coordination, and posture. Yoga, in particular, combines physical postures with mindfulness and controlled breathing, promoting relaxation and reducing stress. The mind-body connection established through flexibility exercises can positively impact cognitive function.

  Interestingly, recent studies indicate that stretching can improve blood glucose regulation, particularly in people with Type 2 diabetes (Thomas et al. 2024). This may be due to changes in the muscle with regular stretching. Combining stretching with mindfulness can be an efficient way to practice both simultaneously, saving you time! We'll discuss mindfulness in more detail later in this chapter.

In addition to these brain and blood glucose benefits, there are other direct brain benefits of physical activity and exercise.

Impact of Exercise and Physical Activity on Brain Health and Neurogenesis

Exercise is known to stimulate the release of neurotrophic factors, such as brain-derived neurotrophic factor (BDNF). These factors support the growth, survival, and function of neurons, fostering a more resilient and adaptable brain. They also play a role in neuroplasticity, which is the brain's ability to reorganize itself and form new connections, contributing to cognitive flexibility (Sleiman et al., 2016).

Regular physical activity has a fascinating impact on the brain's ability to grow new neurons, a process known as neurogenesis. Think of it as the natural way your brain renews itself. When you engage in exercises like walking, running, or even dancing, it triggers a series of events that lead to the creation of fresh neurons (Liu & Nusslock, 2018). These new neurons integrate into existing brain circuits, especially in areas linked to memory and learning, enhancing your brain's plasticity.

So, every time you break a sweat, it's not just your muscles getting stronger; it's your brain getting sharper. The newly formed neurons contribute to improved memory, better learning capabilities, and an overall boost to your cognitive health. It's like giving your brain a refreshing workout, and the benefits extend beyond the gym or the jogging track into your daily life.

Additionally, regular physical activity has been linked to a reduction in inflammation throughout the body, including the brain. Chronic inflammation is associated with various neurodegenerative conditions, and by mitigating this inflammatory response, exercise creates a protective environment for the brain (da Luz Scheffer & Latini, 2020).

By incorporating exercise into your routine, you contribute to the long-term health of your brain, not only boosting your current mental capabilities but creating a shield against conditions like Alzheimer's and age-related cognitive decline.

Incorporating Exercise and Physical Activity into a Regular Routine

- Aim for at least 150 minutes of moderate-intensity exercise per week, such as walking, jogging, or cycling. A guide to moderate intensity, is that you get breathless enough that you can't sing a song, but you can still talk in short phrases.

- Consider brisk walking, a versatile exercise that can be seamlessly integrated into your day. Whether it's a brisk stroll during your lunch breaks, a walk in the park with a friend, walking proves to be a straightforward and impactful choice.

- Cycling to work not only serves as an eco-friendly commute but also contributes to your daily exercise. This dual benefit makes it an efficient way to save time while enhancing fitness.

- Embrace short exercise breaks to combat prolonged sitting and keep your mind refreshed. Standing up, stretching, or engaging in quick exercises every hour can make a notable difference.

- Home workouts provide a convenient solution, often requiring no special equipment. Follow online workout videos, practice bodyweight exercises like squats or push-ups, or use household items for improvised weights.

- Aim to do strength training 2-3 times a week to help you build a regular routine and build or maintain muscle mass.

- Incorporating dance breaks can add an element of fun to your fitness routine! Play your favorite tunes and dance around, turning exercise into an enjoyable and uplifting activity. The key is to find activities that suit your lifestyle and preferences, gradually transforming them into daily habits.

- Be active and regularly move during the day. Non-exercise activity thermogenesis (NEAT) is the concept of energy expended during daily activities and has been linked with improved insulin sensitivity. For example, take the stairs instead of the elevator.

- After-meal gentle movements, such as a gentle walk can help with digestion and stabilize post-meal blood sugar levels, avoiding fluctuations.

- Stretching as a wind-down evening routine not only improves your blood sugar balance, but can also enhance your quality of sleep. We'll cover more about the benefits of sleep next!

Please note that if you have a pre-existing medical condition or on medications, please discuss with your healthcare professional before embarking on a new exercise routine.

Sleep's Role in Glucose Regulation and Brain Health

Did you know that your sleep quality could be influencing not only your energy levels but also the balance of glucose in your body and the health of your brain? There's an important link between getting enough rest, keeping your body's balance, and having a sharp mind.

Sleep Deprivation and Glucose Metabolism

Think back to a night when you couldn't get enough sleep. You likely woke up feeling groggy, a bit off, and maybe even craving an extra cup of coffee. Did you know that this lack of sleep doesn't just make you feel tired but can also mess with how your body handles glucose?

When you don't get enough sleep, it's like throwing a wrench into your body's well-oiled sugar-managing machine. It becomes less efficient at using glucose, and this can lead to problems with thinking clearly and remembering things.

Sleep deprivation can influence insulin sensitivity—with a lack of sleep, your body's cells may become less responsive to insulin. This reduced sensitivity can lead to higher blood sugar levels over time, contributing to insulin resistance, a hallmark of type 2 diabetes.

Additionally, sleep deprivation affects the hormones that regulate appetite. Ghrelin, which stimulates hunger, tends to increase, while leptin, which signals feelings of fullness, decreases. This hormonal imbalance may lead to overeating and poor food choices, further influencing weight gain and the development of diabetes (Grandner et al., 2016). Inadequate sleep can even elevate stress hormones, such as cortisol, which can contribute to insulin resistance and disrupt the body's overall glucose metabolism.

This complex interplay between sleep, hormonal regulation, and insulin sensitivity likely explains the link between insufficient sleep and an increased risk of developing diabetes (Hirotsu et al., 2015).

Circadian Rhythms and Glucose Control

Our bodies operate on a 24-hour internal clock called the circadian rhythm, which influences various biological processes, including sleep-wake cycles, hormone release, and even the way we process glucose. When we maintain a consistent sleep schedule, it allows our circadian rhythm to function optimally and to perform its critical role in glucose regulation.

The circadian rhythm influences the release of hormones like insulin, which helps cells absorb glucose, and cortisol, which plays a role in regulating glucose levels throughout the day. When you stick to a regular sleep pattern, you're aligning the gears of this machine with the natural ebb and flow of your circadian rhythm. This alignment ensures that the release of hormones related to glucose control is synchronized with your body's needs.

Since the brain is highly sensitive to changes in glucose levels, disruptions in glucose regulation can affect cognitive function. By maintaining regular sleep patterns, you are promoting an environment where the circadian rhythm can efficiently coordinate glucose metabolism, supporting not only physical health but also cognitive well-being.

Sleep Quality and Cognitive Recovery

During a night's sleep, your body cycles through different phrases of sleep throughout the night. Each phase has important functions, and quality sleep is important to support cognitive recovery and maintenance.

One of the phases of the sleep cycle is deep sleep. Deep sleep promotes the removal of metabolic waste and toxins that accumulate in the brain throughout the day. This includes substances like beta-amyloid, linked to conditions such as Alzheimer's disease. This is facilitated by the glymphatic system, a waste removal system in the brain that was only recently identified.

Additionally, deep sleep is involved in the regulation of blood glucose levels. During this phase, the body works to maintain optimal glucose

79

metabolism, ensuring that blood sugar remains within a balanced range (Vallet et al., 2023). This process is vital for supporting the brain's energy requirements and promoting cognitive functions.

Impact of Sleep on Willpower and Decision-Making

You know when you're trying to think things through, but it feels like there's a big wall in your brain blocking you from making a decision? Imagine that after a good night's sleep, that wall magically disappears. Your thoughts flow more smoothly, and decisions come to you effortlessly. Quality sleep makes your brain sharper and enhances your decision-making skills, guiding you toward choices that offer lasting benefits.

Sleep deprivation can reduce activity in the pre-frontal lobes of the brain, an area of the brain important for self-control (Pilcher et al., 2015). This could lead to reduced willpower, and increased likelihood of reaching for a sugary snacks.

Strategies for Improving Sleep Quality

Improving sleep quality involves adopting strategies that promote restful and uninterrupted sleep. Here are some practical tips to enhance your sleep:

- **Establish a consistent sleep schedule:** Aim to go to bed and wake up at the same time every day, even on weekends. This helps regulate your body's internal clock.

- **Create a relaxing bedtime routine:** Develop calming pre-sleep rituals, such as reading a book, taking a warm bath, or practicing relaxation exercises. These activities signal to your body that it's time to wind down.

- **Optimize your sleep environment:** Make your bedroom conducive to sleep by keeping it cool, dark, and quiet. Consider blackout curtains, earplugs, or a white noise machine if needed.

- **Limit screen time before bed:** Reduce exposure to screens at least an hour before bedtime. The blue light emitted by devices can interfere with the production of the sleep hormone melatonin.

- **Watch your diet:** Avoid heavy meals, caffeine, and nicotine close to bedtime. These can disrupt rest or make it harder to fall asleep.

- **Stay active during the day:** Regular physical activity can promote better sleep. However, try not to exercise too close to bedtime, as it may energize you.

- **Manage stress:** Practice stress-reducing techniques such as deep breathing, meditation, or mindfulness to ease the mind before bedtime.

- **Limit naps:** If you need to nap, keep it short (20–30 minutes) and limit napping to early afternoon at the latest so as not to affect nighttime sleepiness

- **Evaluate your mattress and pillows:** Ensure your mattress and pillows provide the comfort and support needed for a good night's sleep.

- **Seek professional help if needed:** If persistent sleep problems exist, consider consulting with a healthcare professional or sleep specialist for personalized guidance.

Recognizing and Addressing Sleep Disorders

Recognizing symptoms of sleep disorders, like sleep apnea, is necessary for both brain health and blood glucose regulation. Sleep apnea is a condition where breathing repeatedly stops and starts during sleep. The interruptions in breathing can lead to reduced oxygen levels in the body, affecting various systems. If this happens, seek further assistance from your healthcare professional.

Here are the symptoms to watch out for:

- **Loud snoring**, especially if accompanied by pauses in breathing.

- **Excessive daytime sleepiness** or feeling tired despite a full night's sleep.

- **Morning headaches** result from disrupted sleep patterns.

- **Irritability and mood changes**—sleep disturbances can impact mood.

During sleep, the way we breathe—whether through the mouth or nose—can impact our overall health. Understanding the differences between the two is essential for optimizing sleep quality.

Issues associated with mouth breathing include dry mouth, increased snoring, and disrupted sleep. It may result in less efficient oxygen intake compared to nose breathing and louder snoring due to unregulated airflow. Nose breathing offers advantages such as humidifying and filtering the air and preventing dryness in the respiratory passages. It promotes more controlled and regulated airflow during sleep, enhancing oxygen intake and supporting better overall respiratory function.

Practical Tips for Nose Breathing

- Keep nasal passages clear by using saline sprays or nasal rinses.

- Address issues like allergies or congestion that may hinder effective nose breathing.

- Experiment with sleeping positions that encourage nose breathing.

- Stay adequately hydrated. This helps improve nasal function by keeping the nasal passages moist, preventing dryness and irritation that may cause congestion, discomfort, and difficulty breathing.

- Explore mouth taping. This is a practice where individuals use a gentle adhesive tape to close their lips during sleep to encourage breathing through the nose instead of the mouth. While this practice has gained attention for potentially promoting nose breathing during sleep, ensure that you do not have an underlying nasal problem before attempting it.

You may find it helpful to read my book *Sleep Better To Thrive*, a step-wise guide where I take you through practical strategies to achieve quality sleep. Use this link to access the book: **https://books2read.com/sleepbetter** or search on Amazon.

Mindfulness and Cognitive Function

Now, what exactly is mindfulness? Mindfulness involves paying attention to the present moment without getting lost in worries about the past or future. It's being fully engaged in what you're doing, whether it's eating, walking, or simply sitting quietly.

Just like how regular exercise strengthens muscles, consistent mindfulness meditation seems to fortify specific regions of the brain. Regular mindfulness meditation has been associated with notable changes in the brain's structure. Studies suggest an increase in cortical thickness, especially in areas linked to attention, interoception (awareness of internal body sensations), and sensory processing. These structural changes hold the promise of enhancing memory capacity (Lazar et al., 2005).

But there's more to the story. Mindfulness meditation also plays a role in stress reduction. By engaging in mindful practices, individuals can lower stress levels and decrease the production of cortisol, a hormone that, when elevated, may impair memory and contribute to hippocampus shrinkage. This reduction in stress indirectly supports better memory functionality. In the earlier chapters, we also covered the negative impact of stress on blood sugar regulation.

Mindfulness practices, such as focused breathing and present-moment awareness, contribute to cognitive resilience by enhancing mental adaptability and maintaining optimal brain function in various challenges, including aging and neurodegenerative diseases. Scientific research indicates that regular engagement in mindfulness exercises leads to improved cognitive function with age, acting as cognitive training that preserves mental abilities over time and potentially offering protection against aging processes and neurodegenerative conditions (Sevinc et al., 2021).

Mindfulness in Managing Cravings and Making Healthier Choices

Mindfulness enhances your awareness of bodily sensations and cravings, allowing you to better understand your body's signals and become more attuned to cravings.

Instead of impulsively reacting to a craving, mindfulness can provide the mental space for you to take a pause, and consciously choose how to respond. By being aware of the craving and the sensations associated with it, you gain the ability to respond thoughtfully rather than reactively.

In practical terms, mindfulness helps you distinguish between actual hunger and emotional or habitual cravings, which allows you to make healthier choices. With mindfulness, you're making decisions consciously, ensuring they align with your overall goals.

I am passionate about mindfulness and have dedicated myself to mindfulness teaching and research. I have also written a bestselling book entitled *Mindfulness for Brain Health,* which delves deeper into the practical aspects of incorporating mindfulness into your routine to enhance your cognitive well-being. This link takes you to the book, available in paperback, hardcover, ebook and audiobook: **https://books2read.com/mindfulnessbrainhealth** or you can find it on Amazon.

The Impact of Alcohol and Caffeine on Brain Glucose Levels

For many of us, starting the day with a cup of coffee and winding down with a glass of wine or beer is a common ritual. However, it's crucial to recognize that both caffeine and alcohol can cross the blood-brain barrier and directly influence glucose metabolism in the brain.

Alcohol, Hypoglycemia, and Brain Health

When you consume alcohol, your liver, which is responsible for various metabolic functions, including glucose production, undergoes changes in its normal processes. The liver ordinarily produces and releases glucose into the bloodstream to maintain a stable supply for the body's energy needs. However, alcohol interferes with this process.

This disruption contributes to fluctuations in blood sugar levels, potentially resulting in reduced glucose levels. Hypoglycemia can lead to symptoms like confusion and dizziness and, in severe cases, can even impact consciousness.

Caffeine, Glucose Metabolism, and Cognitive Alertness

Whenever you enjoy a cup of coffee or tea, the caffeine these drinks contain is quickly absorbed into your bloodstream. Caffeine keeps you alert by blocking adenosine in the brain, which is a molecule that makes you feel sleepy.

Additionally, caffeine binds to receptors in the brain that trigger the release of adrenaline. This rush of adrenaline can impact your glucose levels, making your body release some sugar into the bloodstream as a response mechanism. The extra sugar also provides you with a quick energy boost, making you feel more alert and focused.

However, when you have more caffeine than your body needs, it can lead to a surge in adrenaline that results in excess glucose release—and this triggers another response. Insulin goes to work, trying to bring those sugar levels back down to normal. When it succeeds, you might experience a sudden drop in blood sugar, which can leave you feeling jittery, a bit shaky, or even tired. That's why, after the initial high, you might find yourself reaching for another cup of coffee or feeling a bit fatigued.

Additionally, caffeine can affect the quality of your sleep, depending on the timing of consumption. The average quarter-life of caffeine is 12 hours. Let's say you have a cup of coffee at 7 p.m. and intend to go to bed by 11 p.m.—more than a quarter of the amount of caffeine is still in the bloodstream by that time and can affect quality of sleep (Walker, 2017).

Nicotine's Effect on Insulin and Glucose Control

When nicotine enters the body, it triggers a cascade of biological responses. One significant impact is on insulin sensitivity, which, as you know, refers to how well cells respond to the signals of insulin to take in glucose. Nicotine exposure can make cells less responsive to these cues. As a result, glucose uptake becomes less efficient.

It's worth noting that alternatives like e-cigarettes, contain additives that could potentially affect blood sugar levels as well (Górna et al., 2020).

Moderation and Balance in Consumption

You might often hear suggestions like "quit alcohol" or "cut out caffeine," but I get it—making those changes can be tough. It's not as easy as it sounds. However, taking small steps is a key part of reaching a balanced lifestyle.

Let's consider the concept of baby steps—taking gradual, manageable strides toward moderation. Moderation involves finding a middle ground that allows you to enjoy certain aspects while maintaining a balance that supports optimal brain glucose levels and cognitive well-being. It's about understanding the limits and making conscious choices to ensure that these substances do not disrupt the delicate balance of glucose metabolism in the brain.

Embedding new lifestyle changes can be a gradual process. Here are some tips to help you find that balance:

- **Set realistic goals:** Start with achievable goals. Instead of aiming for a complete cut-off, consider reducing your intake gradually.

- **Track your consumption:** Keep a record of how much you're consuming. This helps you become more aware of your habits and allows you to make informed decisions.

- **Designate "no-go" days:** Choose specific days when you'll avoid certain substances. This can create a healthy routine without feeling like you're giving up everything.

- **Alternate with water:** If you enjoy caffeinated or alcoholic beverages, alternate with water. This not only helps with moderation but also keeps you hydrated.

- **Mindful choices:** Before consuming, ask yourself if you genuinely want it or if it's just a habit. Being mindful can help you make conscious decisions.

- **Seek support:** Share your goals with friends or family. Having a support system can make the journey toward moderation more manageable.

- **Educate yourself:** Learn about the effects of these substances on your body and brain. Understanding the impact can motivate you to make healthier choices.

Key Takeaways

This chapter has been a turning point, emphasizing the significant impact of lifestyle habits on our brain health—in addition to diet, as we discussed in the last chapter. Here are five key points to guide you toward optimal cognitive well-being:

- Our daily choices, including exercise, sleep, and mindfulness practices, play a crucial role in shaping the health of our brains. Recognizing this connection is the first step toward improvement.

- Regular physical activity both enhances glucose metabolism and contributes to improved cognitive functions, keeping your brain sharp and resilient.

- Adequate and quality sleep is not just about feeling refreshed; it directly impacts glucose regulation and cognitive recovery. Prioritize those essential hours of shut-eye for overall brain health.

- Mindfulness practices bring about positive changes in brain structure, aiding memory, attention, and emotional regulation. Additionally, mindfulness helps manage cravings and stress, indirectly benefiting blood glucose control and cognitive function.

- Whether it's alcohol or caffeine, moderation is crucial. Small, realistic changes in consumption habits can lead to a healthier balance, supporting optimal brain glucose levels and cognitive health. And if possible, completely eliminate cigarettes.

***

Embark on the next leg of our journey to prime brain health as Chapter 8 explores natural remedies to support your lifestyle choices. This chapter is loaded with insights into herbs and supplements, ranging from ancient remedies to contemporary solutions. Discover the potential impact of these natural offerings on cognitive function and brain glucose levels.

Make a Difference with Your Review

***

Share the Gift of Better Brain Health

"The greatest wealth is health." - Virgil

Congratulations—you're more than halfway through this book! Which parts of this book do you find particularly helpful so far? I hope you don't mind this pause in the book's flow with this little message.

Did you know that sharing knowledge about health can create ripples of positive change throughout our community? Your experience could be the beacon that guides someone else toward better brain health!

Would you help someone just like you—someone who wants to understand their brain better, boost their mental clarity, and take control of their cognitive health, but isn't sure where to start?

My mission is to make the connection between blood sugar and brain health clear and actionable for everyone. But to reach more people who could benefit from this knowledge, I need your help.

Many people rely on reviews when choosing health and wellness books. That's why I'm asking you to help a fellow health-conscious individual by sharing your thoughts in a review.

Taking just a minute of your time to leave a review could help: ...one more professional enhance their mental clarity at work ...one more person overcome their daily energy crashes and mood swings ...one more person clear their persistent brain fog ...one more person live a vibrant life through better understanding of their brain-glucose connection

To share your experience and help others, simply follow the link or scan the QR code to your local Amazon marketplace to leave a review:

USA	UK
Amazon.com/review/create-review?&asin=1917353847	Amazon.co.uk/review/create-review?&asin=1917353847
CANADA	AUSTRALIA
Amazon.ca/review/create-review?&asin= 1917353847	Amazon.com.au/review/create-review?&asin=1917353847

Or search your **Local Amazon Marketplace** and enter
ASIN= 1917353847
or search "Sweet Spot for Brain Health by Dr Sui Wong".

Your review isn't just feedback—it's a helping hand extended to others on their journey to better brain health. Thank you for being part of this mission to improve lives through better understanding of our brain health!   With gratitude, Dr. Sui Wong

Now, let's continue our exploration of the fascinating connection between blood glucose and brain health...

Chapter 8:
Natural Remedies and Supplements

Many of us often overlook the benefits of natural remedies and the potential power of supplements. In this chapter, we focus on the natural supplements that have proven to be beneficial for enhancing brain function and overall cognitive well-being.

Antioxidants and Brain Protection

The brain, constantly active and engaged in various functions, naturally produces reactive oxygen species (ROS) during its processes. In our earlier chapters, we defined ROS as highly reactive molecules containing oxygen that can cause damage to cellular structures. They are natural byproducts of various cellular processes, and while the body has mechanisms to neutralize them, an excess of ROS can lead to oxidative stress, which is associated with various health issues, including inflammation and aging.

As we age, there is a natural and gradual decline in our cognitive function, which can manifest as challenges in memory, reasoning, and other cognitive abilities. This decline is a complex process influenced by various factors, including oxidative stress.

The protective mechanisms of antioxidants involve neutralizing free radicals that can harm cells, including those in the brain. By counteracting oxidative stress, antioxidants may help slow down the deterioration of cognitive function associated with aging.

Moreover, research suggests that antioxidants may have a protective effect against neurodegenerative diseases. Conditions such as Alzheimer's and Parkinson's are characterized by the gradual loss of neurons and cognitive function. Antioxidants, by preventing or reducing oxidative damage to brain cells, may offer a degree of defense against the development and progression of these diseases (Essa et al., 2014).

Antioxidants are abundantly present in various foods and supplements. Including these in your diet can significantly contribute to brain health.

- Berries, like blueberries and strawberries, are packed with antioxidants such as flavonoids and anthocyanins.

- Green tea contains catechins, powerful antioxidants known for their health-promoting properties. Catechins may have neuroprotective effects, supporting the brain's defense against oxidative stress.

- Both vitamin C (ascorbic acid) and vitamin E (tocopherol) are essential antioxidants.

Herbs and Spices for Blood Glucose Control

The use of natural herbs as supplements offers a promising avenue for maintaining stable blood sugar levels. Beyond their impact on blood glucose, some of these herbs also contribute to enhanced brain health. You may wish to consider adding these herbs and spices when you cook.

Cinnamon

Cinnamon, a spice we often use for flavor, does more than just make our food tasty. It can help control blood sugar levels and might have some positive effects on our brains, too. Cinnamon does this by making our cells use glucose efficiently, which is important for managing our blood sugar. It also acts as a supplementary agent to the body's natural insulin functions by imitating insulin and aiding in the cellular uptake of glucose (Qin et al., 2010). This dual action of supporting glucose regulation and mimicking insulin presents an improved approach to blood sugar control.

Apart from helping with blood sugar, cinnamon may also protect the brain. It has special compounds known as cinnamaldehyde that act as shields against stress on our brain cells (Emamghoreishi et al., 2019). Adding cinnamon to your meals is easy. You can sprinkle it on things like rice, cereal, or yogurt, or even mix it into your coffee for extra flavor. But using too much cinnamon could cause other issues, such as coumarin toxicity and liver damage (Raman, 2019).

The two main types of cinnamon are Ceylon and cassia, with cassia being more widely available. Dr. Michael Greger, author of "How Not to Die" and founder of NutritionFacts.org (which provides interesting bite-size nutrition tips), has written an article about the differences between these two types. He suggests using cassia cinnamon for blood sugar regulation and cautions adults not to exceed a teaspoon per day (less for children) due to the compound coumarin in cassia cinnamon (https://nutritionfacts.org/topics/cinnamon/).

Ginseng

Research suggests that ginseng might be good for our pancreas. Ginseng contains bioactive compounds like ginsenosides, which have been studied for their various pharmacological properties. Some studies suggest that these compounds may help regulate blood sugar levels by enhancing insulin sensitivity and secretion from the pancreas (Kochman et al., 2020).

However, it's better to have it earlier in the day and avoid it in the late afternoon or evening. Ginseng can make it harder to fall asleep or stay asleep, on top of causing feelings of restlessness or agitation that can keep you from relaxing and unwinding before bedtime. So, adding ginseng to your routine earlier in the day might be a smart way to support your body's glucose metabolism and potentially benefit your cognitive functions without sacrificing your sleep—which, as we learned in Chapter 7, is also important.

Berberine

Berberine is a natural compound found in various plants, and it has gained attention for its potential benefits in helping the body manage glucose or sugar (Shrivastava et al., 2023). Berberine makes our cells more responsive to insulin. When cells respond well to insulin, it helps maintain balanced blood sugar levels.

Moringa

What makes moringa special are its anti-inflammatory properties and high content of antioxidants, like chlorogenic acid and isothiocyanates. Chlorogenic acid contributes to regulating glucose metabolism and keeping it in balance is essential for overall health (Meng et al., 2013).

Inflammation is linked to various health issues, including those related to diabetes (Rohm et al., 2022). The antioxidants in moringa help combat oxidative stress in our bodies. As we know from previous chapters, managing oxidative stress is crucial, especially in the management of conditions like diabetes where there's an imbalance in the body's antioxidant defense mechanisms.

Omega-3 Fatty Acids and Brain Function

As discussed in Chapter 6, Omega-3 fatty acids play a vital role in supporting both brain function and glucose metabolism. Research suggests that omega-3 supplementation may have various benefits, including improving cognitive function, memory, and concentration.

Additionally, omega-3s act as natural mood boosters and may help alleviate symptoms of depression and anxiety (Wani et al., 2015).

Fortunately, sources of omega-3 are numerous, including several foods you may already eat.

Marine Sources

Fish oil is a rich source of eicosapentaenoic acid (EPA) and DHA, which are long-chain omega-3 fatty acids. These fatty acids are building blocks for our brain cells. Fatty fish like salmon, mackerel, and sardines are rich in these omega-3s. When we consume fish oil, we nourish our brains with a direct supply of the good stuff they need to function properly.

EPA is known for its anti-inflammatory properties. It's like the peacekeeper, helping to calm down any inflammation in the brain. This is crucial because chronic inflammation can be harmful and has been linked to various brain-related issues. DHA is a major structural component of brain cell membranes.

Now, not everyone is a fan of fish, and some people prefer a vegetarian or vegan lifestyle. This is where algae oil comes in. Algae oil is derived directly from algae, which is where fish get their omega-3s from. It's like skipping the middleman and going straight to the source. Just like fish oil, algae oil provides both EPA and DHA, making it an excellent option for vegetarians, vegans, or anyone looking for a plant-based source of these fatty acids.

Plant-Based Sources

Alpha-linolenic acid (ALA) is the omega-3 found in plant-based sources. You can think of it as the starting point, found in foods like flaxseed, chia seeds, walnuts, and hemp seeds. ALA is essential because our bodies can turn it into other important omega-3s, namely EPA and DHA.

- **Flaxseed:** These tiny seeds are packed with ALA. It's like planting the seed for omega-3s in your body. They can be sprinkled on yogurt, added to smoothies, or even used in baking for a boost of ALA.

- **Chia seeds:** Chia seeds are another fantastic source of ALA. They can absorb liquid and turn into a gel-like substance, making them a versatile addition to various dishes.

- **Walnuts:** Walnuts are not just tasty; they're a crunchy source of ALA. It's a snack that not only satisfies your taste buds but also contributes to your omega-3 intake.

- **Hemp seeds:** These little seeds are gaining popularity, and for a good reason. Hemp seeds provide a dose of ALA, contributing to your omega-3 intake.

While ALA is fantastic, the body's ability to turn it into EPA and DHA is a conversion process. Factors like age, sex, and overall health can influence how efficiently this conversion happens. Generally, getting direct sources of EPA and DHA from marine sources, e.g. fatty fish or algae oil, will more directly meet the body's omega-3 needs.

It's also important to note that these plant-based sources are also rich in fiber, supporting a healthy gut microbiome and, in turn, contributing to overall brain health.

Probiotics, Gut Health, and Brain Energy

The gut-brain axis represents the bidirectional communication between the gut (digestive system) and the brain. This connection plays a crucial role in influencing various aspects of our health, including brain function and glucose metabolism.

The gut-brain axis operates through complex interactions involving the nervous system, immune system, and hormones. It enables the gut to send signals to the brain and vice versa, facilitated by the vast network of nerves, the release of chemicals, and the presence of gut microbes.

The composition and activity of the gut microbiota, the community of microorganisms residing in the gut can influence cognitive processes and emotional well-being. A balanced and diverse gut microbiota is associated with positive effects on mood, stress levels, and overall mental health.

Additionally, the gut-brain axis has implications for glucose metabolism—changes in gut health can affect how the body regulates blood sugar levels. This connection is significant, as imbalances in glucose metabolism can contribute to conditions like insulin resistance and diabetes.

Role of Probiotics

Probiotics are live microorganisms, mainly beneficial bacteria and yeast, that can provide health benefits. These microorganisms are often referred to as "good" or "friendly" bacteria because they contribute to the balance of the gut microbiota.

Probiotics can be found in certain foods, such as yogurt, kefir, sauerkraut, and kimchi, as well as in dietary supplements. When ingested, probiotics help maintain a healthy balance of bacteria in the gut, promoting digestive health and potentially offering various other health benefits, including supporting the immune system and influencing brain function. Here are some examples of different probiotics and their reported benefits.

- **Akkermansia muciniphila:** Residing in the mucous layer of the gut, it is known for its ability to regulate gut barrier function. It also plays a role in preventing obesity by improving glucose metabolism and reducing metabolic inflammation (Rodrigues et al., 2022).

- **Lactobacillus and Bifidobacterium strains:** These are known for their ability to improve gut barrier function, reduce inflammation, and potentially alleviate symptoms of anxiety and depression (Kumar et al., 2023). Lactobacillus strains can also help with blood glucose regulation (Chen and Zhang, 2023).

- **Streptococcus thermophilus:** Often used in the production of yogurt and cheese, it aids in breaking down lactose and is beneficial for individuals with lactose intolerance. It also contributes to a healthy gut microbiome (Fijan, 2014).

- **Saccharomyces boulardii:** A yeast probiotic effective in preventing and treating diarrhea, particularly antibiotic-associated diarrhea (Kelesidis & Pothoulakis, 2012). Early studies suggest a potential benefit of this probiotic for metabolic health (Egea et al., 2023).

Glucagon-like peptide 1 (GLP-1) hormone

You may have heard of GLP-1 agonist drugs, a recent class of medication used for glucose control, weight management, and appetite control. Did you know that your own body produces GLP-1? This largely occurs in your gut (Holst, 2007). Natural ways to increase your body's GLP-1 production include maintaining a healthy gut microbiome (Zheng et al., 2024), eating foods high in protein and fiber, and chewing and eating slowly (Fujiwara et al., 2019). The lifestyle factors shared in this book so far also provide the benefit of improving your gut microbiome.

Vitamins for Blood Glucose and Energy Metabolism

Vitamins are essential nutrients that our bodies need to function properly. They are fundamental in various bodily processes, including the way our body uses glucose for energy.

In the process of glucose metabolism, the vitamin B complex is necessary. The B1 vitamin, also known as thiamine, initiates the initial steps of glycolysis, which is essential in the breaking down of glucose.

B3, or niacin, ensures that the energy stored in glucose is released through important metabolic pathways such as glycolysis and the citric acid cycle.

Moving on to B6, or pyridoxine: It is involved in amino acid metabolism, directing these essential building blocks towards energy production. Simultaneously, B12, or cobalamin, is involved in DNA synthesis, nervous system function, and the conversion of fats and proteins into energy.

Biotin, also known as vitamin B7, contributes to glucose metabolism. It acts as a coenzyme for several carboxylase enzymes involved in the metabolism of fatty acids, amino acids, and glucose. One such enzyme is pyruvate carboxylase, which is required for the gluconeogenesis process, where new glucose is formed, helping regulate blood sugar levels (Rodríguez Meléndez, 2000).

Within the metabolic process, the B vitamins function as coenzymes, essential collaborators that facilitate the seamless transformation of nutrients into energy. Their presence is critical for maintaining the balanced and efficient operation of glucose metabolism. The absence of any B vitamin could disrupt this process, leading to an imbalance in energy production. Therefore, the vitamin B complex is essential for ensuring the steady and efficient flow of energy in the complex process of glucose metabolism.

B vitamins are found in a variety of foods including animal proteins, dairy products, leafy green vegetables and beans (Hanna et al., 2022). However, due to the limited vitamin B12 in plant-based diets, vegans are recommended to take vitamin B12 supplements (**https://nutritionfacts.org/topics/vitamin-b12/**).

Minerals for Blood Glucose Control

Minerals are essential nutrients that our bodies need to function properly. These inorganic elements are naturally occurring and can be found in various foods, soil, and water. They are essential for maintaining good health and are involved in a wide range of bodily functions.

The importance of minerals lies in their diverse roles. They contribute to bone and tooth formation, nerve function, fluid balance, and the production of hormones. Additionally, minerals are integral to processes like blood clotting, muscle contraction, and, as we are starting to notice, blood glucose control.

From fruits and vegetables to nuts, seeds, and grains, a balanced diet provides the body with an array of minerals. The following is not a comprehensive list but a highlight of some minerals of particular interest.

- **Magnesium:** Not only does magnesium help directly regulate blood sugar levels, it also aids in the activation of enzymes involved in carbohydrate metabolism, contributing to overall glucose regulation in the body. It can be found in nuts, seeds, whole grains, and leafy green veggies (National Institutes of Health, 2016).

- **Chromium:** Chromium is an important factor for enhancing insulin activity. You can find it in broccoli, potatoes, green beans, and whole-grain goodies (National Institutes of Health, 2017).

- **Zinc:** Zinc is another mineral that supports blood glucose control by participating in insulin storage and release. It is integral to the proper functioning of pancreatic cells, which produce insulin. Adequate zinc levels contribute to the effective regulation of blood sugar. Meat, shellfish, legumes, seeds, and nuts are rich in zinc (Maret, 2017).

- **Selenium:** Selenium is a defender against harm and impacts sugar control. Brazil nuts, seafood, and meats are where you can get your share (National Institutes of Health, 2021).

- **Vanadium:** Vanadium may act like insulin or increase the effects of insulin, helping control glucose. You can find it in small amounts in foods like black pepper, dill, and whole grains (National Library of Medicine, 1999).

- **Calcium:** Calcium is vital for cells, including those making insulin. Dairy, leafy greens, and fortified foods are good sources. (National Institutes of Health, 2022).

Amino Acids and Blood Glucose Regulation

Amino acids serve as an alternative source of glucose when the body faces a shortage. They play a dual role: assisting in muscle building and contributing to blood glucose regulation. By supporting muscle health, amino acids facilitate efficient glucose utilization. Additionally, specific amino acids help maintain stable blood glucose levels by acting as regulators, preventing abrupt spikes or drops.

L-Glutamine

L-Glutamine is an amino acid present in protein-rich foods such as beef, chicken, fish, dairy products, and eggs. Beyond its role in muscle development, L-Glutamine significantly contributes to stabilizing blood glucose levels by influencing insulin regulation and glycogen synthesis (Jafari-Vayghan et al., 2020).

In terms of insulin regulation, L-Glutamine acts as a facilitator, ensuring the timely and coordinated action of insulin. It plays a crucial role in orchestrating insulin's response to maintain glucose balance in the bloodstream. L-Glutamine also contributes to the creation of glycogen, a stored form of glucose. This process ensures a steady supply of glucose when needed, functioning as an energy reserve for the body.

Creatine

Creatine is a substance naturally found in certain foods, like red meat, pork, poultry, and fish. Its primary function revolves around supporting the formation of ATP, a process that proves especially beneficial during short bursts of high-intensity exercise.

When you engage in quick, intense movements, like sprinting or lifting heavy weights, your body requires a rapid burst of energy. This is where creatine steps in, ensuring your muscles have the energy they need for those brief, intense efforts.

Creatine supplementation doesn't just benefit physical performance; it extends its positive influence to cognitive function as well. Research suggests that creatine can enhance memory and executive function, which involves skills like decision-making and problem-solving (Avgerinos et al., 2018).

Interestingly, creatine's positive effects on cognitive function seem to be more noticeable under conditions of sleep deprivation or mental fatigue.

The Downside

While red meat and pork can provide creatine, there are potential downsides to consider.

Firstly, there are sustainability concerns—producing red meat and pork in large quantities can have negative effects on the environment. Additionally, red meat and pork can be high in saturated fat, which, when consumed in excess, could have negative impacts on our heart health.

Moreover, there are ethical concerns related to consuming animal products. For those who prefer not to eat animal products, synthetic creatine supplements are man-made versions of the creatine found in meat that work just as well as getting creatine from meat sources.

Remember to check if the supplement has been third-party tested or has the equivalent of Good Manufacturing Practice certification.

Here are some examples of synthetic creatine supplements (Tinsley, 2017):

- **Creatine monohydrate:** This is the most common and well-researched form of synthetic creatine. It's widely available and known for its effectiveness.

- **Creatine hydrochloride (HCL):** This is another form of creatine that some people find gentler on the stomach compared to creatine monohydrate.

- **Creatine ethyl ester:** This form is believed by some to be more easily absorbed by the body, but scientific evidence supporting this claim is limited.

- **Buffered creatine:** This is creatine monohydrate with an alkaline powder added to reduce its acidity. It's marketed as a way to prevent potential stomach issues.

Key Takeaways

Here, we've explored the often-overlooked world of natural remedies and supplements, emphasizing their potential to support brain health and manage blood glucose levels. Let's recap what we covered so that you can effectively use this information to benefit your daily life:

- Embrace the potential of natural remedies and supplements such as cinnamon, ginseng, berberine, and others.

- Incorporate marine sources like fish or algae oil into your diet for cognitive health and glucose metabolism support.

- Consider including probiotic-rich foods or supplements in your daily routine to promote gut and brain health.

- Ensure adequate intake of vitamin B through foods like eggs, fish, vegetables and beans, to support brain function and energy metabolism.

- Include magnesium-rich foods such as nuts, seeds, whole grains, and leafy green vegetables in your diet to help manage blood sugar levels and support overall health.

***

In Chapter 9, we're going to talk about fasting and how it affects our brains. We'll look into why it's interesting, how it can be good for our cognitive abilities, and how it connects with controlling our blood sugar levels.

Chapter 9:
Fasting and Its Impact on Brain Health

Have you ever considered the idea that fasting could help your brain health? I understand your skepticism; after all, how could depriving your body of food contribute to better brain function when we typically rely on nourishment for survival?

The age-old practice of fasting has demonstrated transformative impacts on cognitive function, metabolic equilibrium, and the activation of autophagy—a natural cellular rejuvenation process.

Understanding Fasting

Fasting is not starvation. Instead, it is a strategic decision to refrain from eating for a certain period, allowing the body to experience a temporary break from the intake of calories. Fasting can take various forms, such as intermittent or time-restricted eating, and prolonged fasting, each with its own unique approach and potential health benefits. In fact, a natural break in eating overnight for 12 hours could be considered a natural form of fasting!

As previously discussed, our bodies typically rely on glucose from carbohydrates for energy. However, in situations when glucose is lacking, there's a metabolic shift from glucose to ketones, which are derived from stored body fat. This transition was explored in detail in the first part of this book. Fasting can help your body adapt to different fuel sources, and therefore improve metabolic flexibility.

When you fast, reduced levels of sugar and insulin prompt your cells to initiate autophagy. Derived from the Greek words "auto," meaning self, and "phagy," meaning eat, autophagy involves the removal and recycling of damaged or dysfunctional cell components. These are then delivered to recycling centers in the cells, called lysosomes, for breakdown into reusable materials.

Now, how does this tie in to our brain health? Fasting may offer benefits such as improved brain energy metabolism, enhanced neuronal plasticity (the brain's ability to adapt and change), and neuroprotective effects. By allowing periods of fasting, it encourages the body to tap into stored energy, promotes cellular repair processes, and may support better brain function.

Fasting and Brain Function

When you're not busy processing food, your body can allocate resources to other important tasks. During fasting, there's a boost in the production of certain chemicals—like brain-derived neurotrophic factor (BDNF), which is vital for forming new memories and improving cognitive functions.

People often report improved focus, better problem-solving abilities, and even a clearer memory during fasting periods (Gudden et al., 2021). Remember, though, that everyone's experience can be a bit different. Some may feel these cognitive benefits more than others, but it's fascinating to see how fasting has the potential to give your brain a boost.

Neuroprotective Impact

When we talk about neuroprotective effects, we mean that fasting might provide a layer of defense against certain brain-related conditions, especially those linked to aging (Zhao et al., 2022). An interesting and evolving idea suggests fasting could offer neuroprotective benefits against conditions like Alzheimer's and Parkinson's disease.

During fasting, your body activates processes that clean up cellular waste and repair damaged components. Additionally, fasting may reduce inflammation by limiting the production of inflammatory signals in the body. Inflammation is often associated with various brain disorders, and by keeping it in check, fasting could be contributing to the overall health and resilience of your brain.

It's important to note that while fasting shows promise in research, it's not a guaranteed shield against these conditions.

Fasting and Blood Glucose Regulation

Intermittent fasting has been shown to enhance insulin sensitivity through several mechanisms. During fasting periods, the body experiences lower levels of circulating glucose, prompting cells to become more receptive to insulin.

Additionally, intermittent fasting promotes the activation of pathways involved in cellular repair and stress resistance, which can improve insulin sensitivity over time. By optimizing insulin sensitivity, intermittent fasting supports better blood sugar control and may reduce the risk of metabolic diseases.

Fasting as a Metabolic Reset

Studies indicate that fasting improves metabolic health, including data showing that long overnight fast can reduce risks for chronic metabolic diseases (Manoogian et al., 2022).

As the body starts utilizing fats for energy, there is a potential for weight loss and a reduction in overall fat mass. This is particularly beneficial for individuals aiming to manage their weight or improve their body composition. The process of breaking down fats for energy is often more sustained and can contribute to a more prolonged sense of energy compared to relying on glucose alone.

Fasting also encourages the development of metabolic flexibility, which refers to the body's ability to adapt to different fuel sources efficiently. In a fasting state, as glycogen stores deplete, the body becomes adept at utilizing not only fats but also ketones, which are byproducts of fat metabolism. This enhanced metabolic flexibility can have positive implications for blood glucose regulation.

The ability to switch between utilizing glucose and fats as primary energy sources provides the body with a more adaptive and resilient metabolic profile. This adaptability is crucial for maintaining stable blood glucose levels, especially during periods of fasting or reduced carbohydrate intake.

How to Fast

If you're considering fasting, you are advised to consult with a healthcare practitioner, especially if you have an underlying medical condition or are on medications.

Importantly for people with a history of eating disorders, please first seek guidance from a healthcare professional, as fasting can trigger disordered eating patterns and risk relapse.

For individuals on diabetic medications, it's crucial to discuss any plans for intermittent or prolonged fasting with your healthcare professional as this may require some adjustments to your medications.

Women who are pregnant and breastfeeding are advised not to fast. If they do so, it should only be under medical guidance.

Intermittent Fasting or Time-Restricted Eating

While a balanced diet focuses on the quality and composition of what we eat, intermittent fasting introduces a different dimension by emphasizing when we eat. It's about adjusting the timing of our meals to match our body's natural rhythms.

The focus is not on restricting the types of food but rather on controlling the timing of meals. During fasting periods, individuals abstain from consuming calories, giving their bodies a break from continuous digestion.

Common methods include the 16/8 method, where one fasts for 16 hours and eats during an eight-hour window (this is also termed "time-restricted eating"), or the 5:2 approach, involving normal eating for five days and significant calorie reduction for two non-consecutive days. Brad Pilon, author of "Eat Stop Eat" and one of the pioneers advocating the benefits of fasting to the public, shares the approach of a 24-hour fast once weekly. For example, starting a fast after breakfast and refraining from any further calories until breakfast the next day. These strategies of a restricted eating window may provide more flexibility with social situations, while promoting various health benefits associated with temporary caloric restriction.

Consider aligning your eating window with the circadian rhythm, matching it with the body's natural rhythms to further enhance the benefits of time-restricted eating (Manoogian et al., 2022).

A suggested approach to start, is to eat within a 10- to 12-hour window linked to daylight hours. In other words, opening your eating window with breakfast in the morning, and closing your eating window after dinner about 10- to 12-hours later. Observe how your body responds, to ease into this safely.

Prolonged Fasting

Prolonged fasting involves extending the fasting period to multiple days, going beyond the shorter durations seen in intermittent fasting or time-restricted eating. This approach aims to induce more profound effects on the body. It is recommended that this approach is done under medical guidance. Following medical guidance and listening to your body's needs is especially crucial when taking part in prolonged fasting that's practiced over several days.

Personalized Responses to Fasting

We are all unique, and our bodies exhibit distinct responses to various stimuli, including fasting. How one person responds to a fasting regimen may differ significantly from another. Factors such as genetics, overall health, lifestyle, and existing metabolic conditions help shape individual responses.

Some individuals may experience more stable blood glucose levels during fasting, while others might encounter fluctuations. It's essential to recognize and appreciate this variability. What works well for one person might not yield the same results for another.

This underscores the importance of adopting personalized approaches to fasting. Rather than adhering strictly to a one-size-fits-all model, individuals should consider tailoring their fasting practices to align with their unique needs and responses. Personalization might involve adjusting the duration and frequency of fasting periods or incorporating specific dietary considerations.

Monitoring is key in this process. Regular tracking of blood glucose levels, energy levels, and overall well-being can provide valuable insights into how an individual's body is responding to fasting. This data-driven approach allows for adjustments and refinements, ensuring that fasting practices align optimally with an individual's health goals.

However, it's essential to consider the potential impact of prolonged fasting on lean muscle mass, which is pivotal for maintaining insulin sensitivity and promoting healthy aging. Therefore, it's important to incorporate strategies to preserve lean muscle mass while engaging in fasting practices, such as ensuring adequate protein intake, and incorporating resistance training exercises into your routine. By prioritizing the preservation of lean muscle mass, you can optimize your fasting experience while supporting long-term health outcomes.

Practical Tips for Fasting

Now that you've understood the potential benefits of fasting to improve your brain health and metabolic flexibility, you may wish to start fasting. If so, here are some practical tips to help you ease into fasting.

- **Start gradually**. It may be best to start off with time-restricted eating. For example, if your current eating window is from 6am to 10pm (16 hours), start by reducing your eating window to 14 hours (e.g. 6am to 8pm). As you adapt, gradually reduce your eating window until you reach your initial target of 12 hours (e.g. 7am to 7pm). If you wish to continue to build on this, slowly reduce the eating window until you reach your next target, e.g. 10 hours.

- **Start your fast after an early dinner** (e.g. 5-6 pm) and breaking fast in the morning. This way, you'll be sleeping through a significant portion of your fasting period. Having an early dinner will also allow time for your body to digest food and avoid it affecting your sleep. Breaking fast in the morning also helps align with your circadian rhythm.

- **Plan your fasting schedule around your social life**. It's okay to be flexible and adjust your fasting times for special occasions or social events.

- **Keep hydrated when fasting**. Drink regular sips of water throughout the day. Hot cups of non-calorific tea or coffee can be helpful. These should be non-calorific, i.e. with no sugar, cream, or fats.

- **Avoid artificial sweeteners** during your fast as this may trick your body into thinking you are consuming sugar, which can affect your metabolic regulation. Even zero-calorie drinks can potentially trigger an insulin response.

- **Break your fast with low-to-moderate glycemic index or glycemic load foods**. This is to avoid sharp swings in blood sugar. For example, break your fast with vegetables and protein.

- **During your eating window, continue to practice healthy eating habits** (e.g. what we covered in Chapter 6). Remember that intermittent fasting is not a license to eat junk food or over-eat during your eating window!

- **When you get food cravings**, notice if this is due to physical hunger or if it is a habit or response to emotion.

- **Do regular strength training** to maintain your muscle mass and avoid excessive muscle loss from fasting. Brad Pilon who I mentioned earlier, shared the strategy of an "anabolic fast" where one starts fasting after a strength training session and a protein-rich meal.

- **Eating sufficient protein during your eating window to maintain muscle mass**. Protein needs vary, with recommendations ranging from 0.8 to 1.7 grams of protein per kilogram of body weight. For a starting guide and calculator, visit this Harvard Medical School resource: https://www.health.harvard.edu/blog/how-much-protein-do-you-need-every-day-201506188096

- **Consider tracking your fasts using a mobile app**. This can help you monitor your progress and stay motivated.

- **Be patient with yourself**. It may take time for your body to adapt to fasting. Don't get discouraged if you don't see immediate results.

- **Listen to your body**. If you feel unwell during a fast, it's okay to break it. Fasting should make you feel better, not worse. If you feel lightheaded during a fast, check if this is could be due to excessively low blood sugar levels (hypoglycemia) or low blood sugar – seek assistance from a healthcare professional.

- **If fasting starts to trigger disordered eating, pause and reflect if this is serving you and your health**. Discuss this with a healthcare practitioner.

- **Remember that fasting is a form of stress on the body**. Consider how much stress your body is currently experiencing, and whether it is the right time to fast. For example, if someone is in the middle of starting a new job, juggling care of a young family and elderly parents, or training for a marathon, adding fasting to the mix may be too much stress for the body.

- As stated previously, remember to **consult a healthcare professional** before starting any fasting regimen, especially if you have a pre-existing health condition or on medications.

Key Takeaways

In this chapter, we delved into the transformative effects of fasting on brain health and blood glucose regulation. Fasting, an ancient practice, was explored in various forms, including intermittent fasting or time-restricted eating, and prolonged fasting. We examined the physiological changes during fasting, as well as its cognitive enhancements, neuroprotective benefits, and its role in improving insulin sensitivity and blood glucose regulation. Furthermore, the concept of fasting as a metabolic reset and its potential effects on autophagy for brain health were thoroughly discussed.

- Fasting comes in various forms and each approach offers unique benefits for brain health and overall well-being.

- Fasting triggers a shift from glucose to ketone metabolism, promoting efficiency in burning stored fats. This metabolic flexibility aids in regulating blood glucose levels.

- Fasting has the potential to enhance cognitive functions such as memory, focus, and problem-solving abilities. It may act as a natural cognitive booster.

- Fasting might offer neuroprotective benefits, lowering the risk of neurodegenerative diseases like Alzheimer's and Parkinson's. The removal of damaged cells during autophagy plays a crucial role.

- Individual responses to fasting vary. Understanding one's body and adopting a personalized approach to fasting is essential for optimizing its benefits.

***

Our next chapter will unravel secrets on how to overcome challenges you may face as you improve and maintain your brain health, ensuring you can stay motivated.

Chapter 10:
Overcoming Challenges and Staying Motivated

As we embark on this journey to optimize brain health, setbacks may arise, testing our resilience. Think about a time when you've encountered a challenge. You may have felt a bit scared at first, maybe even overwhelmed. Conquering challenges isn't easy. The fear and anxiety they inspire can quickly take over, causing us to procrastinate every attempt at working through the obstacle. Sometimes, you have to allow yourself to be scared as you face a challenge.

Don't try to do it all at once, either. This only makes the process more difficult. Instead, take small steps every day. When you're working to improve and nurture your brain health, these small steps add up over time and provide you with more valuable benefits. In this chapter, we're going to take a look at how you can overcome challenges and stay motivated, as well as tips you could implement to ensure your journey to better brain health is a success.

Stress Management and Blood Glucose Control

One of the most common challenges you will face throughout your life is stress. Stress comes in many forms—from the stress you experience at work to stressing about finding time to go grocery shopping or visit a friend for their birthday during a busy week. Different types of stress will also affect you in different ways, impacting you on a physical, mental, and emotional level.

In Chapter 4, we learned that stress can influence blood sugar, and blood sugar can affect your stress levels. This is important to keep in mind because stress experienced for long periods can lead to a consistently high amount of sugar in your bloodstream. While the rapid burst of energy this provides you with is valuable during a single stressful moment, it can quickly become overwhelming when you're constantly experiencing stress. This is when you will benefit from stress management techniques.

Throughout this book, we've discussed several strategies and activities that will help you care for your brain health and manage your blood glucose, and we've also looked at how you can incorporate stress management techniques. As such, you're already familiar with many of the strategies available to you.

However, the management technique that works for one person won't always work for you. You may even find that specific techniques only work during certain situations. For example, a mindful breathing activity might help you handle unexpected events at work, but physical activity may work better for helping you reduce your overall stress. This means that you need to experiment with the different strategies to figure out which ones work best for you.

You could even make a list that you can keep on your phone or in a notebook. When you notice yourself starting to feel stressed out or overwhelmed, take out your notes and choose one of the strategies that help you. Remember that the activity should suit the environment you're in and meet your needs at that moment. For example, taking out your yoga mat for a 10-minute relaxation routine might not be suitable for an office environment. Instead, you could try deep breathing, progressive muscle relaxation (PMR), or even take a short walk in the fresh air before sitting down at your desk again.

There's no right or wrong way to do this either since everyone is so different. But you can draw from common stress management techniques to help you create a plan that meets your needs and suits your lifestyle. In the list that follows, you'll find a few examples of how to incorporate the activities we've already discussed in previous chapters:

- **Mindfulness:** Mindful breathing can be practiced while you get ready for work or as you sit down in front of your computer. You could also use mindful eating practices while drinking your morning cup of tea or coffee, or even while you eat lunch.

- **Deep-breathing exercises:** This activity is great for combating feelings of overwhelm and can easily be practiced anywhere.

When you notice that you're starting to feel as though the stress is too much, find a quiet space (this could be your office, the bench outside, your bedroom, or even your car). Once you've found your spot, inhale deeply through your nose, hold your breath briefly, and exhale slowly through your mouth. Repeat this process several times.

- **Meditation:** Meditation doesn't mean you have to sit cross-legged on a yoga mat. You can meditate while having a cup of tea at a local café, walking in the park, or even sitting in your office or the break room at work. While you're seated, focus on your breath or a chosen point of attention, and allow your mind to become still. If you're walking or doing a repetitive activity, simply shift your focus to the task and allow yourself to become immersed in it.

- **Yoga:** Yoga is great for practicing breath control, immersing yourself in physical movement, meditating, and even burning off extra energy. This is an activity that is typically better suited to home or a group class, but if you don't have time for a long session, you could practice a 10-minute yoga stretching routine or just do a few simple poses. There are several yoga resources available online. The one you choose to use should meet your needs.

- **Progressive muscle relaxation (PMR):** This technique involves systematically tensing and relaxing different muscle groups, promoting a sense of calm. Start with your toes and work your way up through the body, tensing and then releasing each muscle group. What's so great about this activity is that you can practice it anywhere, at any time.

You may be interested in my book *Mindfulness for Brain Health*, which includes free mindfulness meditation audioguides. The book shares practical strategies for self-care and stress management. You can access this book via this link: **https://books2read.com/mindfulnessbrainhealth** or search the Amazon store.

Harnessing Technology for Health Management

In the current era, we have the remarkable opportunity to enhance various aspects of our lives through technology. Studies suggest that mobile health (mHealth) apps have the potential to alleviate symptoms, and contribute to overall health restoration (An et al., 2023).

Health apps can be versatile tools for the management of blood glucose levels. For example, apps for dietary tracking to monitor food intake, track macronutrients, and maintain a comprehensive record of meals. By having a clear overview of your dietary habits, you can make informed choices to align your eating patterns with your blood glucose goals.

There are also apps to monitor physical activity, logging various exercises, track steps, and gauge overall physical exertion. Maintaining an awareness of physical activity levels is crucial for managing blood glucose effectively, as regular exercise positively influences insulin sensitivity and overall metabolic health.

Incorporating these apps into your routine can enhance your ability to proactively manage blood glucose levels and promote a resilient approach to health. Tap into this potential power of mobile health apps by searching your app store for relevant apps based on your goals and what you would like to track.

Checklists for Success

The following are some checklists to consider as you move forward to build a plan for success. You could also use this alongside the bonus 12-Week Challenge in the Appendix.

Creating a Personalized Action Plan

Planning is essential for success, and setting achievable goals tailored to our unique needs is key. This involves creating realistic objectives that consider our health status, daily routines, and preferences. For example, goals may focus on dietary changes, exercise, and lifestyle adjustments, all personalized to suit individual circumstances. Personalized goal-setting ensures sustainability and motivation, guiding us towards better blood glucose management over the long term.

For example, I had a patient who was grappling with high cholesterol levels, and upon further investigation, we found that fluctuating blood glucose levels played a significant role as part of their metabolic health dysregulation. By making simple yet impactful changes, such as incorporating more beans and pulses into their diet and engaging in well-timed exercise like taking a walk after meals, we observed improvements not only in their blood glucose but also in their cholesterol levels. This experience underscores the importance of personalized interventions, including goal-oriented dietary adjustments and strategic physical activity, for comprehensive health improvement.

Incorporating Personal Preferences and Routines

For a plan to be successful, it has to align with your unique preferences and routines, making the journey both effective and enjoyable. It's about creating health-conscious habits that resonate with your lifestyle, ensuring a successful and personalized health adventure. In the previous chapters, we covered many lifestyle approaches that can improve blood sugar balance for better brain and metabolic health. Which ones would you like to start with? Some examples are as follows, which we covered in previous chapters.

- **Smart snacking:** Choose snacks wisely. Opt for nutrient-dense options like nuts, yogurt, or fresh fruits. These choices not only support your health but also contribute to stable blood glucose levels.

- **Routine-friendly exercises:** Incorporate physical activity into your routine. Whether it's a short walk after meals or quick exercises at home, finding activities you enjoy ensures regularity. You'll be surprised by what a daily evening stroll can do for your health.

- **Mindful eating practices:** Practice mindful eating by savoring each bite. This not only enhances your dining experience but also aids in recognizing and responding to your body's hunger and fullness cues.

Regular Review and Adaptation of the Plan

Reflecting on our health goals is essential to ensure they remain realistic and achievable. Goal reassessment allows us to modify objectives based on our evolving needs and circumstances. Our routines and preferences may change over time. Adapting the plan to align with these changes keeps it sustainable and enjoyable, so you'll feel more motivated to stick to it.

- **Routine check-ins:** Regularly assess how your body responds to the current plan. Are there any positive changes? Any unexpected challenges? Keep a diary to track daily observations.

- **Health professional consultations:** Schedule periodic discussions with healthcare professionals. Their insights can provide a deeper understanding of your health status and guide necessary adjustments.

- **Goal reassessment:** Reflect on your initial health goals. Have you achieved them, or do they need modification? Setting realistic and achievable goals is a continuous process.

- **Lifestyle and preferences:** Life is dynamic, and so are our routines and preferences. Adapt your plan to align with changes in your daily life and evolving tastes.

- **New research:** Stay informed about the latest health research. New findings may offer insights into refining your plan for better outcomes.

- **Social support:** Engage with support groups or communities. Sharing experiences and tips with others managing blood glucose can provide valuable perspectives.

Dealing with Setbacks and Maintaining Resilience

Facing setbacks in blood glucose management is a common part of the journey, but it's imperative to approach them with resilience and a mindset of growth. Here are some simplified strategies to help you recognize setbacks and turn them into opportunities for learning and improvement:

- **Acknowledgment:** Recognize that setbacks happen to everyone. It's not a sign of failure but an indication that adjustments may be needed.

- **Reflective journaling:** Keep a simple journal to note patterns and circumstances surrounding setbacks. This can help identify triggers and guide future decisions.

- **Learning opportunities:** View setbacks as opportunities to learn more about your body and its responses. Understanding what didn't work allows you to refine your approach.

- **Seeking support:** Reach out to your healthcare team, friends, or support groups. Sharing experiences and gaining different perspectives can offer valuable advice and encouragement.

- **Small adjustments:** Instead of overhauling your entire plan, consider small, manageable adjustments. Gradual changes are often more sustainable and easier to incorporate.

Building Resilience and Staying Motivated

Building resilience in managing blood glucose involves adopting positive coping strategies and maintaining long-term motivation.

Building Resilience

- **Positive outlook:** Cultivate a positive mindset. Focus on what you can control rather than dwelling on challenges. Recognize that setbacks are temporary and part of the journey.

- **Self-compassion:** Be kind to yourself. Acknowledge that managing blood glucose is a continuous process, and it's okay to face difficulties. Treat yourself with the same kindness you would offer a friend.

- **Mindfulness:** Practice mindfulness to stay present and reduce stress. Techniques like deep breathing or meditation can enhance emotional well-being and resilience.

- **Adaptability:** Embrace flexibility. Understand that adjustments to your plan may be necessary. Being adaptable helps in navigating unexpected situations.

Staying Motivated

- **Celebrate small victories:** Acknowledge and celebrate every achievement, no matter how small. Recognizing progress, even minor, reinforces a sense of accomplishment.

- **Set new challenges:** Keep motivation alive by setting new, realistic challenges. It could be trying a healthy recipe, increasing physical activity gradually, or achieving stable blood glucose levels for a specific period.

- **Visualize long-term goals:** Remind yourself of the bigger picture. Visualize the long-term benefits of managing blood glucose—improved health, increased energy, and a better quality of life.

- **Personalized rewards:** Establish a system of personalized rewards for reaching milestones. These can be non-food-related treats that align with your interests, providing positive reinforcement.

- **Reflection:** Regularly reflect on your journey. Consider how far you've come, lessons learned, and the positive impact on your overall well-being. This reflection enhances motivation.

Social Support and Accountability

Building a strong social network is a powerful asset in the journey of managing blood glucose levels for better brain health. Positive social connections are more than just heartwarming; they're stress-busters pivotal for your brain's well-being. When you engage in positive social interactions, the stress response in your body tends to diminish. Sharing light moments with your peers could be all you need to overcome the stress that has been mounting on your health.

Stress, if left unchecked, can wreak havoc on both your brain health and your blood glucose levels. However, a robust social network acts as a buffer, mitigating the impact of stressors. Think of it as having friends and loved ones who share the load, making the journey through life's challenges a bit lighter.

- **Community strength:** Foster an environment of support within your family and friend circles. Share your health goals and challenges openly, allowing others to contribute positively.

- **Support groups:** Participate in support groups focused on blood glucose management. These communities provide a platform for shared experiences, advice, and motivation.

- **Family involvement:** Ensure your family understands the importance of blood glucose management for brain health. Educate them on healthy lifestyle choices and involve them in your journey. Engage in activities that promote a healthy lifestyle together. This could include cooking nutritious meals, going for walks, or participating in wellness activities as a family.

- **Friendships:** Communicate your health goals to close friends. Having friends who understand and support your objectives creates a positive peer influence. Plan social outings that involve physical activities, promoting a healthy and active lifestyle.

- **Accountability partners:** Team up with someone who shares similar health goals. Establish similar commitments and regularly check in on each other's progress. Celebrate milestones together, reinforcing the sense of accomplishment and shared success.

- **Peer pressure:** Positive health behaviors within your social circle can create a norm, and the desire to adhere to these norms serves as motivation. Jointly pursuing health goals with friends or family provides a shared goal, making the journey more enjoyable and sustainable.

- **Joining clubs:** Consider joining clubs or community organizations aligned with your interests. Whether it's a book club, a sports team, a gardening group, or a community service organization, shared activities provide a natural setting for forming bonds with like-minded individuals.

- **Volunteering opportunities:** Engaging in volunteer work not only benefits your community but also opens avenues for meeting new people who share your passion for making a positive impact. It's a meaningful way to connect with others while contributing to a greater cause.

- **Group exercises or classes:** Participating in group exercises or classes, such as fitness classes, dance lessons, or art workshops, not only promotes physical well-being but also fosters social interaction. The shared experience of learning or exercising together can lead to lasting connections.

- **Maintaining regular contact:** In our fast-paced lives, maintaining regular contact with friends and family can sometimes take a backseat. However, prioritizing quality interactions over quantity is key. A heartfelt conversation, even if infrequent, can strengthen relationships.

Key Takeaways

Be proud of the path you are taking and your commitment toward a healthy life! Here are a few takeaways from this chapter to carry along:

- Regularly review and adjust your action plan based on changing health needs and circumstances.

- Like any journey, setbacks are normal. Learn from them, adapt, and continue forward.

- Leverage the support and resources available through online communities for motivation.

- Incorporate individualized goal-setting to ensure realistic and achievable milestones.

***

Learning to overcome challenges on any health journey is an important part of your success, but you might be wondering how you can cultivate a lifestyle that helps you continuously nurture your brain's health. In the next chapter, we'll explore some of the best ways to remain consistent on our journey, as well as techniques to successfully incorporate what we've learned from this book into our daily lives.

Chapter 11:
Staying on Top of Brain Health

In this final chapter, we consolidate our learnings and delve deeper into comprehensive approaches for nurturing lifelong brain health. From the importance of cognitive exercises and regular health check-ups to the transformative potential of collaborative care, we explore how a multifaceted approach can pave the way for enduring cognitive resilience and well-being.

The Role of Regular Health Check-Ups

Monitoring blood glucose levels is not just a routine task; it's a profound investment in your overall well-being, with a direct impact on your brain health. As you've learned throughout this book, your brain relies heavily on a steady supply of glucose for optimal function.

Fluctuations in glucose levels, if left unchecked, can contribute to cognitive decline and increase the risk of neurodegenerative diseases. By staying vigilant, you empower yourself to identify and address these fluctuations promptly, paving the way for sustained mental clarity, focus, and overall cognitive resilience.

For individuals managing diabetes, consistent monitoring provides real-time data that guides treatment decisions, helping you strike the delicate balance needed to keep your blood glucose within a healthy range. This tailored approach safeguards against immediate risks while laying the foundation for a lifestyle that promotes enduring brain health.

Comprehensive Health Assessments for Preventive Care

In the quest to preserve brain health, regular physical exams and screenings enable the early detection and management of conditions that could jeopardize cognitive function.

Routine checks include vital signs, blood tests, and tailored screenings offer personalized insights, enabling healthcare providers to identify specific risk factors and offer recommendations to individual profiles. This approach forms the foundation for a brain-healthy lifestyle, ensuring timely and precise preventive measures aligned with individual health needs.

Collaborative Care Approach

In my many years as a medical professional, I have valued the power of collaborative healthcare. This strategy involves forming a dedicated team that goes beyond healthcare providers to include nutritionists, psychologists, and fitness experts. Together, this interdisciplinary team works cohesively to craft a holistic plan personalized to your unique needs.

Your healthcare provider plays a central role, overseeing your medical condition and coordinating with other specialists. A nutritionist contributes insights into dietary choices that support stable blood glucose levels and promote brain health. A psychologist can be a valuable source of support for emotional and mental wellbeing. A fitness expert provides guidance on physical activities that align with both your overall health and cognitive well-being.

Brain Training and Cognitive Exercises

This book's focus has been on the importance of blood sugar regulation and metabolic health for your brain and wellbeing. Nevertheless, it is helpful to be reminded of these additional measures to support your brain health.

The brain is a dynamic and flexible organ that thrives on challenges and new experiences. Learning and experiencing new things stimulates various regions of your brain, encouraging the formation of new neural pathways and strengthening existing ones. This process is known as neuroplasticity, and it's a lifelong process that can support our brain health. But what's the best way to encourage this activity regardless of your lifestyle? Continuous learning.

Just like physical exercise is vital for the body, mental exercise is crucial for the brain. Embracing new challenges, being curious, and engaging in activities that push the boundaries of our knowledge contribute to the health and vitality of our brains throughout our lives.

Cognitive Exercises for Brain Stimulation

Engaging in cognitive exercises is like a workout for the brain, helping to keep it sharp and agile. These activities stimulate various cognitive functions, promoting mental acuity and preserving cognitive abilities. Here are some examples of exercises that you can incorporate into your routine:

- **Puzzles and brainteasers:** Sudoku, crossword puzzles, and jigsaw puzzles challenge your problem-solving skills and memory. These activities require you to think critically, strategize, and recall information, which can help keep your mind sharp and agile. Plus, they offer a fun and enjoyable way to challenge yourself and keep your brain engaged.

- **Memory games:** Play memory card games or try recalling lists of items to enhance your memory. These activities are specifically designed to improve your retention and recall abilities. By regularly practicing memory games, you can strengthen your cognitive functions and enhance your overall mental acuity.

- **Language learning:** Language learning is a stimulating activity that engages various cognitive functions and promotes brain health. Whether you choose to learn through language learning apps, enroll in classes, or explore online resources, immersing yourself in a new language provides numerous benefits. It not only enhances your linguistic abilities but also stimulates different areas of the brain involved in memory, attention, and problem-solving.

- **Reading and discussions**: Read books and articles to enrich your knowledge and understanding of various subjects. Engage in discussions with others to exchange viewpoints and insights, stimulating critical thinking and expanding your understanding of the world.

- **Mindfulness and meditation:** Practices that promote mindfulness and meditation can improve focus, concentration, and overall cognitive well-being.

- **Critical thinking exercises:** These involve solving problems, analyzing situations, and engaging in activities that challenge your cognitive abilities. By actively questioning, evaluating, and synthesizing information, you can enhance your analytical skills and develop a more nuanced understanding of complex concepts. These exercises encourage you to think critically, consider multiple perspectives, and make informed decisions, ultimately sharpening your problem-solving abilities and fostering intellectual growth.

- **Learning a musical instrument:** Playing an instrument involves coordination, memory, and concentration, providing a holistic brain workout that enhances cognitive abilities and promotes overall brain health.

- **Learning movement:** Activities like dance or tai chi train the brain's center for motor coordination, enhancing cognitive functions related to balance, coordination, and spatial awareness.

Adding Cognitive Activities to Your Daily Routine

Enhancing cognitive health doesn't require a major overhaul of your schedule. Here are some practical and easy ways to seamlessly integrate cognitive activities into your life:

- Discover a multitude of mobile applications specifically crafted to provide a wide array of cognitive exercises and games. These innovative apps offer quick and enjoyable challenges, ideal for short breaks, ensuring entertaining mental stimulation throughout your day.

- Participate in clubs or groups centered on shared interests or learning. Whether it's joining a book club, language exchange group, or any community that encourages mental stimulation, these engagements foster growth and intellectual development.

- Immerse yourself in creative hobbies such as painting, writing, or crafting, allowing your imagination to flourish and your artistic side to thrive. These activities serve as more than just outlets for self-expression; they also activate various regions of the brain, fostering creativity, problem-solving skills, and cognitive flexibility.

- Dedicate a specific time each day to immerse yourself in reading. Whether you're captivated by the imaginative realms of fiction or drawn to the informative depths of non-fiction, regular reading offers a gateway to diverse ideas and perspectives. Engaging with various genres and subjects not only enriches your knowledge but also stimulates your intellect and fosters a deeper understanding of the world around you.

- Incorporate mindfulness into your daily routines by fully immersing yourself in each activity. Whether you're cooking a meal, tidying up your space, or taking a leisurely stroll, strive to be present and attentive. Mindfulness cultivates heightened focus and mental clarity, enriching your experience of each moment.

- Enhance your knowledge by tuning in to educational podcasts during your commute or workout sessions. This convenient practice enables you to effortlessly absorb new information and expand your understanding of various topics.

- Maximize your productivity by multitasking with intention. For instance, consider listening to an audiobook or educational podcast while engaging in household chores. This way, you can efficiently complete tasks while also absorbing valuable knowledge and information. This not only makes mundane activities more engaging but also allows you to make the most of your time by combining leisure with productivity.

Key Takeaways

From the importance of cognitive exercises to the significance of lifelong learning and social engagement, we discussed actionable strategies for maintaining cognitive wellness. Recognizing the vital role of comprehensive health assessments and collaborative care, the chapter emphasized the holistic approach required for sustaining brain health and blood glucose stability.

- Embracing a mindset of continuous learning and engaging in cognitive exercises supports neuroplasticity, contributing to improved memory, learning, and cognitive function.

- Regular monitoring of blood glucose levels is imperative, especially for individuals at risk of or managing diabetes, to ensure early detection and effective management.

- Consider a collaborative care approach involving healthcare professionals, nutritionists, and fitness experts to create a personalized and holistic plan for brain wellness.

Conclusion

Together, we've explored the fascinating world of nutrition, cognitive function, and the pivotal role blood glucose plays in sustaining our brain health. Throughout these chapters, we've explored the complexities of maintaining stable blood glucose levels, uncovering the profound impact it has on cognitive vitality.

Consider this book not just as a guide but as a companion on your ongoing quest for a healthier, more vibrant life. Feel free to revisit its pages, extract new gems of wisdom, and reinforce the valuable lessons you've acquired.

Remember, knowledge is a living entity—it grows as you apply it. Implement the strategies, embrace the lifestyle changes, and let your journey to optimal brain health be a continuous exploration. As we bid adieu, stay curious, stay informed, and stay committed to your well-being. The path to a healthier, sharper mind is an ongoing process—one that you are now well-equipped to navigate. Your dedication to learning and evolving is a testament to your commitment to a vibrant and fulfilling life.

I'd like to kindly ask for a moment of your time. If you found value in the insights, strategies, and knowledge shared in this book, I would greatly appreciate it if you could leave a review. Your thoughts and feedback are invaluable, and I'll read all your comments and reviews. They not only inspire me to continue creating content that matters but also help fellow readers make informed decisions about their reading choices. Your review is a small gesture that can make a big impact.

May your journey toward cognitive vitality be as enriching as the knowledge you've gathered within these pages. Here's to your health, your mind, and the incredible journey that lies ahead.

***

In this book we covered about the importance of Sleep and Mindfulness as powerful tools for your blood sugar balance and brain health. You can access my books on these topics using these links or searching on Amazon

Sleep Better to Thrive: **https://books2read.com/sleepbetter**

Mindfulness for Brain Health: **https://books2read.com/mindfulnessbrainhealth**

***

Have you enjoyed this book and would like to be updated on my future book releases?

Receive news about my upcoming books, and get my Thursday Tips [TT] where I share bite-size brain health tips to thrive, via **bit.ly/drwongbrainhealth**

Follow me on Amazon Author Central to receive alerts on new upcoming books! **https://www.amazon.com/author/drsuiwong**

Keeping the Knowledge Flowing

Now you have everything you need to understand your brain-glucose connection and optimize your cognitive health, it's time to share this vital knowledge with others who are looking for answers.

Simply by leaving your honest opinion of this book on Amazon, you'll help guide other health-conscious individuals toward better understanding of their brain health. Your review could be the beacon that leads someone else to discover how they can enhance their mental clarity, overcome brain fog, and take control of their cognitive wellbeing.

Thank you for your help. The journey to better brain health becomes easier when we share our discoveries with others – and you're helping me reach more people who want to understand and optimize their brain-glucose connection.

Simply leave a review using the link or QR code to your Amazon marketplace

USA	UK
Amazon.com/review/create-review?&asin=1917353847	Amazon.co.uk/review/create-review?&asin=1917353847
Or search your **Local Amazon Marketplace** and enter ASIN= 1917353847 or search "Sweet Spot for Brain Health by Dr Sui Wong".	

With gratitude, Dr Sui Wong

Appendix

Book Bonuses: Would you like a copy of my favorite chickpea snack recipe, mentioned in Chapter 6? Request it using this link: **bit.ly/sweetspotbonuses**

Thursday Tips! Get my popular Thursday Tips [TT] where I share bite-size brain health tips to thrive – a 1-min read with 3 tips and 1 question! – sign up via **bit.ly/drwongbrainhealth**

Get alerts on upcoming book releases, via **bit.ly/drwongbrainhealth**

SCAN ME

Other books you may enjoy:

These books by Dr Wong may be of interest, and are available on Amazon as paperback, e-book, and audiobook:

Sleep Better to Thrive: **https://books2read.com/sleepbetter**

Mindfulness for Brain Health: **https://books2read.com/mindfulnessbrainhealth**

Quit Ultra-Processed Foods Now: **https://books2read.com/quitupf**

Bonus:
12-Week Challenge

Throughout this book, we've covered a variety of strategies for improving your brain health and ensuring its long-term well-being. In this bonus chapter, you will find a 12-week challenge to guide you in your journey. This challenge contains additional activities and tips to help you continue pursuing optimal brain health.

Putting Knowledge into Action

Now that you've gained valuable insight into various aspects of brain health, nutrition, and well-being, it's time to put that knowledge into action. This 12-week challenge consists of interactive exercises designed to help you actively apply the lessons learned throughout the book. So how does it work?

Every week, you're going to take one exercise and work through it at your own pace. For example, exercise 1 will be practiced on week 1, exercise 2 on week 2, and so on. By giving yourself a week to work through each activity, you have time to determine the best way to approach it, as well as how you can incorporate it into your life. Remember that healthy habits take time to build. This challenge gives you the foundation needed to be successful and remain consistent.

While you may feel a bit overwhelmed at first, the following tips can help you ensure your success:

- Use a journal to keep track of your progress and make notes on the activity you're working on for that week.

- Record any challenges you face while working on the exercise. These could be mental, physical, or emotional challenges.

- Be sure to record your successes as well, no matter how small. It's also a good idea to take time to celebrate your success each week. Remember that your success doesn't have to be recognized by the whole world to matter.

- At the end of every challenge, reflect on the exercise. It may be a good idea to record your thoughts so you can note what methods worked best for you and how you fit the activity into your unique lifestyle.

- Additionally, write down how you might approach the exercise and fit it into your daily schedule the next time you practice it.

- If you struggle to remain consistent when working on challenges, consider doing the challenge with a trusted friend or family member. That way, you can support each other, work on the challenges together, and hold each other accountable.

Before you get started on the first activity, remind yourself that you don't need to complete the exercise in a single day. Small steps add up. So be patient with yourself and work slowly through each activity to maximize the benefits you stand to gain. Let's get started with the first activity.

Exercise 1: Keep a Food Diary

- **Start your diary:** Begin by setting up a simple food diary. You can use a notebook, a smartphone app, or even a spreadsheet to track your meals and snacks.

- **Record everything:** For one week, diligently record everything you eat and drink throughout the day. Be sure to include portion sizes and note the carbohydrate content of each item.

- **Analyze your choices:** At the end of the week, review your food diary. Take note of patterns in your eating habits and how they correlate with your energy levels and mood.

- **Reflect and learn:** Reflect on how different types of carbohydrates, such as simple sugars versus complex carbohydrates, may have influenced your blood glucose levels and cognitive function.

- **Identify areas for improvement:** Identify any areas where you could make healthier food choices or better manage your carbohydrate intake to support sustained energy and mood stability.

Tips for Success

- Be honest and thorough in your recording to get an accurate picture of your dietary habits.

- Consider seeking guidance from a nutritionist or dietitian for personalized insights based on your food diary findings.

Exercise 2: Mindful Eating

- **Select your meal:** Pick one meal per day to practice mindful eating. Opt for any mealtime that fits into your daily routine.

- **Preparation:** Prior to beginning your meal, pause for a moment to observe the visual presentation, aroma, and texture of your food. Engage all your senses.

- **Eat slowly:** As you commence eating, adopt a leisurely pace. Chew your food deliberately and attentively, focusing on the flavors and sensations with each bite.

- **Tune into taste:** Be fully present as you consume your meal. Notice how each morsel tastes and the sensations it evokes in your mouth. Pay attention to the interplay of flavors and textures.

- **Monitor energy and clarity:** Throughout the meal, be mindful of any shifts in your energy levels and mental clarity. Take note of any changes in how you feel before and after eating.

- **Reflect:** Upon completing your meal, take a moment to reflect on your experience. Consider how the mindful eating practice influenced your enjoyment of the meal and your overall well-being.

- **Consistent practice:** Aim to integrate mindful eating into your daily routine. With regular practice, you can cultivate a deeper connection to your food and enhance your awareness of bodily signals.

Tips for Success

- Minimize distractions during your mindful eating sessions to fully immerse yourself in the experience.

- Experiment with various food choices to explore different tastes and textures.

Exercise 3: Brain-Boosting Meal Plan

- **Week-long meal planning:** Dedicate time to plan a week's worth of meals and snacks tailored to support optimal brain function.

- **Nutrient balance:** Ensure each meal incorporates a balanced mix of complex carbohydrates, healthy fats, and lean proteins to provide sustained energy for your brain.

- **Variety and exploration:** Experiment with diverse recipes and ingredients to discover combinations that enhance cognitive performance and keep you alert and focused throughout the day.

- **Mindful selection:** Mindfully select foods known for their brain-boosting properties, such as leafy greens, fatty fish rich in omega-3 fatty acids, nuts and seeds, whole grains, and antioxidant-rich fruits and vegetables.

- **Portion control:** Practice portion control to avoid overeating and maintain stable blood glucose levels, which are essential for optimal brain function.

- **Adapt and adjust:** Be flexible with your meal plan and willing to adjust based on your energy levels, dietary preferences, and nutritional needs.

Tips for Success

- Incorporate brain-boosting ingredients like turmeric, blueberries, avocados, and dark chocolate into your recipes.

- Experiment with meal timing and frequency to determine what works best for your energy levels and cognitive performance.

- Keep a journal to track how different foods and meal combinations impact your mood, energy, and focus throughout the week.

Exercise 4: Label Reading Challenge

- **Grocery store exploration:** Allocate a specific time during your next grocery shopping trip to focus on reading food labels.

- **Identify hidden ingredients:** Carefully examine the labels of packaged foods to identify sources of added sugars, refined carbohydrates, and other artificial additives.

- **Whole food selection:** Prioritize choosing whole foods and minimally processed options over heavily processed products.

Look for foods that are rich in nutrients, fiber, and essential vitamins and minerals.

- **Sugar awareness:** Pay close attention to the various names used for added sugars, including sucrose, high fructose corn syrup, dextrose, and maltose, among others. Be cautious of products marketed as "low-fat" or "diet," as they often contain added sugars to enhance flavor.

- **Carbohydrate consideration:** Evaluate the carbohydrate content of foods, focusing on complex carbohydrates from sources like whole grains, fruits, and vegetables rather than simple sugars and refined carbohydrates.

- **Glycemic impact:** Consider the glycemic index (GI) of foods, which measures how quickly carbohydrates in food raise blood glucose levels. Aim for foods with a lower GI to prevent rapid spikes and crashes in blood sugar.

- **Read food labels thoroughly:** Take your time to read and understand the entire ingredient list and nutritional information panel on food labels. Look for foods with minimal ingredients and avoid products with lengthy lists of artificial additives and preservatives.

Exercise 5: Physical Activity Routine

- **Routine development:** Dedicate time to create a personalized exercise routine tailored to your fitness level and preferences. Incorporate a combination of aerobic exercises, such as brisk walking, cycling, or swimming, and strength-training activities like weightlifting or bodyweight exercises.

- **Frequency and duration:** Aim for at least 30 minutes of moderate-intensity exercise most days of the week. Schedule your workouts at times that align with your daily routine and energy levels, whether it's in the morning, during lunch breaks, or in the evening.

- **Variety and enjoyment:** Keep your exercise routine diverse and enjoyable by incorporating different activities and workout formats. Experiment with outdoor activities, group fitness classes, or home-based workouts to keep motivation high and prevent boredom.

- **Mindful movement:** During your workouts, pay attention to how physical activity affects your body and mind. Notice changes in your energy levels, mood, and cognitive function before, during, and after exercise sessions.

- **Progress tracking:** Keep track of your physical activity habits and progress over time. Use a fitness journal, smartphone app, or wearable fitness tracker to monitor your workouts, record achievements, and set new goals.

Tips for Success

- Start with achievable goals that align with your current fitness level and schedule. Gradually increase the intensity, duration, and frequency of your workouts as you progress.

- Experiment with different types of physical activity until you find ones that you genuinely enjoy. Whether it's dancing, hiking, or playing a sport, incorporating activities you love into your routine will make exercise more enjoyable and sustainable.

- Treat exercise like any other appointment by scheduling it into your daily or weekly calendar. Consistency is key to developing a lasting exercise habit, so commit to regular workout times that work for you.

Exercise 6: Stress Management Techniques

Exploring stress-relief practices: Experiment with various stress-reduction techniques to discover which ones resonate most with you. Some popular options include:

- **Deep breathing:** Practice diaphragmatic breathing exercises to activate the body's relaxation response and calm your nervous system.

- **Meditation:** Engage in mindfulness meditation or guided meditation sessions to cultivate awareness, presence, and inner peace.

- **Yoga:** Incorporate yoga into your routine to promote physical flexibility, mental relaxation, and stress relief through gentle movements, breathing exercises, and meditation.

- **Progressive muscle relaxation:** Learn to systematically tense and release muscle groups throughout your body to promote physical relaxation and alleviate tension.

- **Nature walks:** Spend time outdoors in nature, whether it's a leisurely stroll through the park or a hike in the wilderness, to reduce stress and improve mood.

Creating your stress-relief routine: Once you've explored different stress-relief practices, choose one or more techniques to incorporate into your daily routine. Consistency is key to reaping the benefits of stress management, so aim to practice your chosen techniques regularly, ideally every day.

Observing the impact: As you integrate stress-relief practices into your daily life, pay close attention to how they affect your overall well-being. Notice any changes in your mood, energy levels, physical sensations, and cognitive function before, during, and after engaging in stress-management activities. Keep a journal to track your experiences and reflect on the effectiveness of different techniques.

Exercise 7: Sleep Hygiene Checklist

- **Establish a consistent bedtime routine:** Set a regular sleep schedule by going to bed and waking up at the same time each day, even on weekends. This helps regulate your body's internal clock and promotes better sleep quality.

- **Create a sleep-friendly environment:** Make your bedroom conducive to sleep by keeping it cool, dark, and quiet. Invest in a comfortable mattress and pillows, and consider using blackout curtains or white noise machines to block out any distractions.

- **Limit screen time before bed:** Minimize exposure to screens from electronic devices such as smartphones, tablets, and computers at least an hour before bedtime. The blue light emitted by these devices can disrupt your body's natural sleep-wake cycle and make it harder to fall asleep.

- **Practice relaxation techniques:** Wind down before bed with relaxation techniques such as deep breathing exercises, gentle stretching, meditation, or reading a book. Avoid engaging in stimulating activities or stressful tasks close to bedtime.

- **Watch your diet and hydration:** Avoid consuming large meals, caffeine, or alcohol close to bedtime, as these can interfere with your ability to fall asleep and stay asleep. Opt for light, nutritious snacks if you're hungry before bed, and stay hydrated throughout the day to prevent nighttime awakenings due to thirst.

- **Manage stress and anxiety:** Address any underlying stress or anxiety that may be affecting your ability to sleep. Practice stress-relief techniques such as mindfulness, journaling, or talking to a trusted friend or therapist to promote relaxation and peace of mind before bedtime.

- **Track your sleep patterns:** Keep a sleep journal or use a sleep tracking app to monitor your sleep quality and duration each night. Note any factors that may affect your sleep, such as caffeine intake, exercise, or stressful events, and make adjustments to your sleep routine as needed.

Exercise 8: Blood Glucose Monitoring

- This exercise is for people who have, or are suspected to have, blood sugar disorders. Please discuss this with your healthcare professional.

- **Select a blood glucose meter:** Choose a reliable blood glucose meter that fits your needs and preferences. Consult with your healthcare provider or pharmacist for recommendations on meter selection and usage.

- **Establish testing times:** Determine specific times of the day to test your blood sugar levels, such as before meals, after meals, before and after exercise, and before bedtime. Testing at different times provides valuable insights into how your blood glucose fluctuates throughout the day.

- **Keep a detailed log:** Record your blood glucose readings in a logbook or a digital app, along with relevant information such as the time of day, corresponding meals or snacks, physical activity, medication intake, and any symptoms or feelings you experience.

- **Identify patterns:** Review your blood glucose log regularly to identify patterns and trends. Pay attention to how different foods, meal timing, exercise routines, stress levels, and other factors influence your blood sugar levels. Look for patterns of highs and lows and consider factors that may contribute to these fluctuations.

- **Make adjustments:** Use the insights gained from monitoring your blood glucose levels to make informed decisions about your diet, exercise, medication, and lifestyle habits. Work with your healthcare team to develop personalized strategies for managing your blood sugar levels and optimizing your overall health.

Exercise 9: Hydration Challenge

- **Calculate your water intake goal:** Determine your daily water intake goal based on your body weight and activity level. As a general guideline, aim to drink at least 8 glasses (64 ounces) of water per day, but adjust this amount based on factors such as your weight, age, gender, climate, and physical activity level.

- **Stay hydrated throughout the day:** Keep a reusable water bottle with you wherever you go to ensure easy access to water throughout the day. Set reminders on your phone or use hydration tracking apps to prompt you to drink water regularly, especially if you have a busy schedule or tend to forget to hydrate.

- **Listen to your body:** Pay attention to your body's signals for thirst and dehydration. Drink water whenever you feel thirsty, and be mindful of other signs of dehydration such as dry mouth, dark urine, fatigue, dizziness, or headaches. If you engage in physical activity, spend time outdoors in hot weather, or consume caffeinated or alcoholic beverages, you may need to increase your fluid intake to stay adequately hydrated.

- **Monitor your fluid intake:** Keep track of your daily water intake using a hydration journal or a hydration tracking app. Note the quantity of water you consume throughout the day, as well as any other fluids such as herbal tea, infused water, or electrolyte beverages. Aim to spread your fluid intake evenly throughout the day rather than consuming large amounts all at once. A helpful rule-of-thumb is to aim for straw-colored urine.

- **Choose hydrating foods:** Incorporate hydrating foods with high water content into your diet, such as fruits (e.g., watermelon, oranges, strawberries), vegetables (e.g., cucumbers, lettuce, celery), soups, and broth-based dishes. These foods can contribute to your overall fluid intake and provide additional nutrients and hydration benefits.

- **Adjust for individual needs:** Adjust your water intake based on individual factors such as your level of physical activity, exposure to hot or humid weather, medical conditions, medications, and pregnancy or breastfeeding status. Consult with a healthcare professional if you have specific concerns or medical conditions that may affect your hydration needs.

Daily Water Tracker

- **Monday:**

- **Tuesday:**

- **Wednesday:**

- **Thursday:**

- **Friday:**

- **Saturday:**

- **Sunday:**

Exercise 10: Brain-Boosting Recipe Swap

- **Curate your brain-boosting recipes:** Begin by selecting your favorite brain-healthy recipes that feature ingredients known to support cognitive function and overall brain health. Look for recipes rich in nutrients like omega-3 fatty acids, antioxidants, vitamins, and minerals. Consider dishes that incorporate brain-friendly ingredients such as leafy greens (e.g., spinach, kale), fatty fish (e.g., salmon, mackerel), nuts and seeds (e.g., walnuts, flaxseeds), whole grains, and colorful fruits and vegetables.

- **Share and exchange:** Reach out to friends, family members, or colleagues who share your interest in cooking and wellness. Invite them to participate in the recipe swap challenge by exchanging their own favorite brain-boosting recipes. You can communicate through social media, email, or in-person gatherings to facilitate the exchange of culinary inspiration.

- **Experiment and explore:** Embrace the opportunity to explore new flavors, ingredients, and cooking techniques as you try out the recipes shared by your peers. Challenge yourself to step out of your culinary comfort zone and experiment with diverse cuisines and cooking styles. Take note of the unique flavors, textures, and nutritional benefits of each recipe you prepare.

- **Cook and share together:** Organize cooking sessions or potluck gatherings where you and your fellow participants can cook, taste, and enjoy the brain-boosting dishes together. Create a supportive and collaborative cooking environment where everyone can contribute their culinary creations and share their cooking tips, experiences, and feedback.

- **Document and celebrate:** Document your recipe swap journey by taking photos of the dishes you prepare and sharing them with the group. Share your cooking successes, challenges, and discoveries along the way. Celebrate the joy of cooking and eating delicious, nutrient-rich meals that nourish both body and mind.

- **Reflect and learn:** Reflect on how incorporating brain-healthy recipes into your diet impacts your overall well-being, energy levels, mood, and cognitive function. Pay attention to any positive changes you experience in terms of mental clarity, focus, and overall vitality. Use this experience as an opportunity to learn more about the connection between nutrition and brain health.

Exercise 11: Brain Training Games

- **Select your brain training platform:** Begin by choosing a reputable brain training app or accessing online resources that offer a variety of cognitive exercises and games designed to challenge and improve different aspects of brain function. Look for platforms that offer a diverse range of activities, including puzzles, memory games, problem-solving tasks, and language exercises.

- **Set daily goals:** Establish a daily goal for your brain training sessions, aiming to dedicate at least 15 minutes each day to engage in cognitive exercises. Set aside a specific time during your day when you can focus on your brain training activities, whether it's in the morning before starting your day, during a break, or in the evening as a relaxing wind-down activity.

- **Choose a variety of challenges:** Explore the different types of cognitive exercises available on your chosen platform and select a variety of challenges to keep your brain engaged and stimulated. Mix and match activities that target different cognitive domains, such as attention, memory, problem-solving, and language skills, to provide a comprehensive workout for your brain.

- **Track your progress:** Keep track of your performance and progress over time by monitoring your scores, completion times, and improvement trends across various brain training activities. Many brain training apps provide built-in features that allow you to track your progress and visualize your improvement through detailed performance metrics and analytics.

- **Stay consistent and persistent:** Commit to maintaining a consistent brain training routine, incorporating it into your daily schedule as a regular habit. Consistency is key to reaping the long-term benefits of brain training, so make an effort to prioritize your cognitive health and stick to your daily practice, even on busy days or when faced with other commitments.

- **Challenge yourself and have fun:** Approach your brain training sessions with a positive and curious mindset, embracing the challenge of tackling new and progressively more difficult tasks. Challenge yourself to push beyond your comfort zone and continuously strive for improvement while also enjoying the process and having fun with the games and activities.

Exercise 12: Staying Consistent Even When You Don't Want To

Knowing how to take care of your brain health is important, but you might find it overwhelming to consistently incorporate the strategies you've been provided into your daily life. You may even struggle to choose a specific activity. In this exercise, you're going to build a plan to help you implement the knowledge you've gained and combat any boredom that may arise from practicing the same activity over again.

Step 1: The Activity List

In addition to the activities in this chapter, we've explored a variety of techniques throughout this book that will help you improve the health of your body and mind. In a notebook, compile a list of these activities. Be sure to add any activities that you've found helpful. It may even be useful to note how this activity helped you (one or two sentences will work).

Now that you have your list, you're going to separate the activities into categories. You may even add additional activities like daily habits, sleep habits, and any challenges you want to work on. I've provided examples of three possible categories here:

- **Daily habits:** Any habit that you practice every day, like taking medication or vitamins, eating, drinking water, and sleeping. If you have a specific routine for a habit (eating could involve meal-prepping activities and grocery shopping, while sleep habits include a nighttime routine), write it down as well.

- **Exercise habits:** Note the physical activities you enjoy taking part in. If you have specific routines revolving around exercise (like stretching or listening to a podcast while exercising), include this.

- **Hobbies:** It's important to make time for the things you care about. This may include going to a dance class, painting, knitting, or even learning an instrument.

- **Brain care:** Activities like doing puzzles, learning about something you're interested in, going to museums, or reading, for example, would fall into this category.

Step 2: The Timebound Table

In this step, we will determine the time restrictions for the activities we categorized in Step 1. This helps you decide which activities deserve your immediate attention, as well as which can be completed when time permits.

Start by taking the list of activities from the previous step (which were separated into categories) and placing them into the following timebound table.

Take note that the activities in this table will change every week as your schedule changes. After all, your friend's birthday isn't a weekly event and you may have done enough grocery shopping and meal prepping for two weeks and don't need to do so this week. So be sure to adjust the table accordingly.

Timebound: Short	Important activities that either need your attention every day or that have a deadline. For example, waking up at 6:30 a.m. every morning and going on a morning walk at 7 a.m.
Timebound: Medium	Any activity that is important but not urgent. This could include making time for grocery shopping and meal prepping. Even mental health activities like journaling may be considered important.
Timebound: Long	Activities that aren't urgent, but will need your attention within the next week or month. This would include making time for hobbies and brain-training games.
Timebound: As time permits	Activities you'd like to do as time permits. The label reading challenge or swapping out your recipes for new ones are examples of this.

Remember that this table will change each week and should *only* contain activities that you will be focusing on for that specific week. Cycling through activities is important because it allows you to choose exercises that you enjoy and that meet your energy requirements and schedule.

Step 3: The Weekly Schedule

You will then create your schedule for the week using the two previous steps. Keep in mind that it's important to set aside time to take care of different activities. Consider putting a time limit on them to help you. It's also helpful to write down any weekly goals you may have so that you can give them attention.

For example, you could aim to exercise three times a week for 30 minutes. You could also set boundaries like limiting your screen time to only a few hours every day. But be sure to replace a habit like this one with a different one, like working on a brain puzzle instead.

You can now use the weekly schedule table to arrange your days. Instead of just filling in work activities, you will block out time for the activities from the timebound table. Try to avoid overwhelming yourself, too. You don't need to do every activity in a single day or week. I've provided an example of what this might look like in the table below. However, you can approach the table in any way that you feel comfortable with.

Monday	To-Do for the Day:
Wake up at 7 a.m.	Make an appointment for the next check-up.
Mindfulness meditation	
Breakfast	
Take medication	
Work	
Dinner	
Start my new mystery novel	
Tuesday	**To-Do for the Day:**
Wake up at 7 a.m.	Call Grandma and ask her about her trip.
Journaling activity	
Breakfast	
Take medication	
Work	
Dinner	
Me time	

Wednesday	To-Do for the Day:
Wake up at 7 a.m.	
Yoga	
Breakfast	
Take medication	
Work	
Dinner	
Family dinner at 7 p.m.	
Thursday	**To-Do for the Day:**
Wake up at 7 a.m.	Errands
Morning off	
Breakfast	
Take medication	
Work	
Music lesson at 6:30 p.m.	
Dinner	

Friday	To-Do for the Day:
Wake up at 7 a.m.	Laundry
Brain training activity: Crossword puzzle	
Breakfast	
Take medication	
Work	
Dinner	
Painting	
Saturday	**To-Do for the Day:**
Wake up at 7 a.m.	
Breakfast	
Take medication	
Hiking with Ruby at 8 a.m.	
Early lunch at 11 a.m.	
Meal planning at 2 p.m.	
Game night with friends at 6 p.m.—bring snacks	

Sunday	To-Do for the Day:
Wake up at 7 a.m.	Plan for the week ahead
Breakfast	
Take medication	
Grocery shopping at 11 a.m.	
Meal preparation from 2 p.m. to 4 p.m.	
Movie night	

Tips for Success

If you're working on a specific goal, like improving your sleep, you could break the activity down into smaller, easier-to-achieve steps that would either be included in your schedule, or kept as a separate list you could easily refer to when needed. These steps should set out exactly what needs to be done and by when. For example:

- Waking up every morning at the same time, like 6 a.m.

- Have a morning routine, like making your bed immediately after waking, doing a light stretching routine, and then getting ready for the day, for example.

- In the evenings, aim to finish working three hours before bed so that you can practice a mental wind-down routine. This may include working on a relaxing hobby or turning on dimmer lighting.

References

The references provided here include a mixture of scientific articles and websites that provide valuable information and that you can easily access to do further reading. Keep in mind that new studies are constantly being conducted. You can use the resources here to help you build your knowledge base and take your health journey into your own hands.

Ajimera, R. (2020, June 2). *Glycemic index: What it is and how to use it.* Healthline. https://www.healthline.com/nutrition/glycemic-index#what-it-is

Altayyar, M., Nasser, J. A., Thomopoulos, D., & Bruneau, M. (2022). The implication of physiological ketosis on the cognitive brain: A narrative review. *Nutrients, 14*(3), 513. https://doi.org/10.3390/nu14030513

An, Q., Kelley, M. M., Hanners, A., & Yen, P.-Y. (2023). Sustainable development for mobile health applications using the human-centered design process (preprint). *JMIR Formative Research.* https://doi.org/10.2196/45694

Attia, P., & Gifford, B. (2023). *Outlive: The Science and Art of Longevity.* Vermilion.

Avgerinos, K. I., Spyrou, N., Bougioukas, K. I., & Kapogiannis, D. (2018). Effects of creatine supplementation on cognitive function of healthy individuals: A systematic review of randomized controlled trials. *Experimental Gerontology, 108*, 166–173. https://doi.org/10.1016/j.exger.2018.04.013

Beard, E., Lengacher, S., & Dias, S. (2021). *Astrocytes as key regulators of brain energy metabolism: New therapeutic perspectives. 12.*

https://www.frontiersin.org/articles/10.3389/fphys.2021.8258
16/full

Cacciatore, M., Grasso, E. A., Tripodi, R., & Chiarelli, F. (2022). Impact of glucose metabolism on the developing brain. *Frontiers in Endocrinology, 13*. https://doi.org/10.3389/fendo.2022.1047545

Calkin, C. V., Gardner, D. M., Ransom, T., & Alda, M. (2013). The relationship between bipolar disorder and type 2 diabetes: More than just co-morbid disorders. *Annals of Medicine, 45*(2), 171–181. https://doi.org/10.3109/07853890.2012.687835

CDC. (2022, May 21). *The effects of diabetes on the brain.* Centers for Disease Control and Prevention. https://www.cdc.gov/diabetes/library/features/diabetes-and-your-brain.html

Chen S, Zhang Y. (2023). Mechanism and application of *Lactobacillus* in type 2 diabetes-associated periodontitis. *Front Public Health.* 30;11:1248518. doi: 10.3389/fpubh.2023.1248518.

Chia, C. W., Egan, J. M., & Ferrucci, L. (2018). Age-Related changes in glucose metabolism, hyperglycemia, and cardiovascular risk. *Circulation Research, 123*(7), 886–904. https://doi.org/10.1161/circresaha.118.312806

Clapp, M., Aurora, N., Herrera, L., Bhatia, M., Wilen, E., & Wakefield, S. (2017). Gut microbiota's effect on mental health: The gut-brain axis. *Clinics and Practice, 7*(4). https://www.ncbi.nlm.nih.gov/pmc/articles/PMC5641835/

Continuous glucose monitoring. (n.d.). National Institute of Diabetes and Digestive and Kidney Diseases. https://www.niddk.nih.gov/health-information/diabetes/overview/managing-diabetes/continuous-glucose-monitoring

Corinne O'Keefe Osborn. (2017, June 27). *How to recognize and manage a blood sugar spike.* Healthline; Healthline Media. https://www.healthline.com/health/blood-sugar-spike

da Luz Scheffer, D., & Latini, A. (2020). Exercise-induced immune system response: Anti-inflammatory status on peripheral and central organs. *Biochimica et Biophysica Acta. Molecular Basis of Disease,* *1866*(10). https://doi.org/10.1016/j.bbadis.2020.165823

de la Monte, S. M., & Wands, J. R. (2008). Alzheimer's disease is type 3 diabetes—evidence reviewed. *Journal of Diabetes Science and Technology,* *2*(6), 1101–1113. https://doi.org/10.1177/193229680800200619

Deshpande, O. A., & Mohiuddin, S. S. (2020). *Biochemistry, oxidative phophorylation.* PubMed; StatPearls Publishing. https://www.ncbi.nlm.nih.gov/books/NBK553192/

Duelli, R., & Kuschinsky, W. (2001). Brain glucose transporters: Relationship to local energy demand. *Physiology, 16*(2), 71–76. https://doi.org/10.1152/physiologyonline.2001.16.2.71

Edwards, S. (2016). *Sugar and the Brain.* Hms.harvard.edu; Harvard Medical School. https://hms.harvard.edu/news-events/publications-archive/brain/sugar-brain

Egea MB, Oliveira Filho JG, Lemes AC (2023). Investigating the Efficacy of *Saccharomyces boulardii* in Metabolic Syndrome Treatment: A Narrative Review of What Is Known So Far. *Int J Mol Sci*, 24(15):12015. doi: 10.3390/ijms241512015.

Emamghoreishi, M., Farrokhi, M. R., Amiri, A., & Keshavarz, M. (2019). The neuroprotective mechanism of cinnamaldehyde against amyloid-β in neuronal SHSY5Y cell line: The role of n-methyl-d-aspartate, ryanodine, and adenosine receptors and glycogen synthase kinase-3β. *Avicenna Journal of Phytomedicine*, 9(3), 271–280. https://www.ncbi.nlm.nih.gov/pmc/articles/PMC6526042/

Essa, M., Al-Adawi, S., Memon, M., Manivasagam, T., Akbar, M., & Subash, S. (2014). Neuroprotective effects of berry fruits on neurodegenerative diseases. *Neural Regeneration Research*, 9(16), 1557. https://doi.org/10.4103/1673-5374.139483

Fijan, S. (2014). Microorganisms with claimed probiotic properties: an overview of recent literature. *International Journal of Environmental Research and Public Health*, 11(5), 4745–4767. https://doi.org/10.3390/ijerph110504745

Freeman, A. M., & Pennings, N. (2019). *Insulin resistance*. Nih.gov; StatPearls Publishing. https://www.ncbi.nlm.nih.gov/books/NBK507839/

Fujiwara Y, Eguchi S, Murayama H, Takahashi Y, Toda M, Imai K, Tsuda K. (2019). Relationship between diet/exercise and pharmacotherapy to enhance the GLP-1 levels in type 2 diabetes. Endocrinol Diabetes Metab. 2(3):e00068. doi: 10.1002/edm2.68.

Gomez-Virgilio, L., Maria-del-Carmen Silva-Lucero, Diego-Salvador Flores-Morelos, Gallardo-Nieto, J., Lopez-Toledo, G., Arminda-Mercedes Abarca-Fernandez, Zacapala-Gómez, A. E., José Luna-Muñoz, F. Montiel-Sosa, Soto-Rojas, L. O., Mar Pacheco-Herrero, & Maria-del-Carmen Cardenas-Aguayo. (2022). *Autophagy: A key regulator of homeostasis and disease: An overview of molecular mechanisms and modulators.* *11*(15), 2262–2262. https://doi.org/10.3390/cells11152262

Górna, I., Napierala, M., & Florek, E. (2020). Electronic cigarette use and metabolic syndrome development: A critical review. *Toxics*, *8*(4), 105. https://doi.org/10.3390/toxics8040105

Goyal, M. S., & Raichle, M. E. (2018). Glucose requirements of the developing human brain. *Journal of Pediatric Gastroenterology and Nutrition*, *66*, S46–S49. https://doi.org/10.1097/mpg.0000000000001875

Grandner, M. A., Seixas, A., Shetty, S., & Shenoy, S. (2016). Sleep duration and diabetes risk: Population trends and potential mechanisms. *Current Diabetes Reports*, *16*(11). https://doi.org/10.1007/s11892-016-0805-8

Gudden, J., Arias Vasquez, A., & Bloemendaal, M. (2021). The effects of intermittent fasting on brain and cognitive function. *Nutrients*, *13*(9), 3166. https://doi.org/10.3390/nu13093166

Harris, R. A., & Harper, E. T. (2015). Glycolytic pathway. *ELS*, 1–8. https://doi.org/10.1002/9780470015902.a0000619.pub3

Hirotsu, C., Tufik, S., & Andersen, M. L. (2015). Interactions between sleep, stress, and metabolism: From physiological to pathological conditions. *Sleep Science*, *8*(3), 143–152. https://doi.org/10.1016/j.slsci.2015.09.002

Holland, K. (2018, May 9). *The connection between sugar and depression.* Healthline; Healthline Media.

https://www.healthline.com/health/depression/sugar-and-depression#carbohydrates-and-depression

Holst JJ. (2007). The physiology of glucagon-like peptide 1. Physiol Rev. 87(4):1409-39. doi: 10.1152/physrev.00034.2006.

Jafari-Vayghan, H., Varshosaz, P., Hajizadeh-Sharafabad, F., Razmi, H. R., Amirpour, M., Tavakoli-Rouzbehani, O. M., Alizadeh, M., & Maleki, V. (2020). A comprehensive insight into the effect of glutamine supplementation on metabolic variables in diabetes mellitus: a systematic review. *Nutrition & Metabolism*, *17*(1). https://doi.org/10.1186/s12986-020-00503-6

Jena, A. B., Samal, R. R., Bhol, N. K., & Duttaroy, A. K. (2023). Cellular red-ox system in health and disease: The latest update. *Biomedicine & Pharmacotherapy*, *162*, 114606. https://doi.org/10.1016/j.biopha.2023.114606

Jessen, N. A., Munk, A. S. F., Lundgaard, I., & Nedergaard, M. (2015). The glymphatic system: A beginner's guide. *Neurochemical Research*, *40*(12), 2583–2599. https://doi.org/10.1007/s11064-015-1581-6

Kay, I. (2019, October 21). *Is your mood disorder a symptom of unstable blood sugar?* Sph.umich.edu. https://sph.umich.edu/pursuit/2019posts/mood-blood-sugar-kujawski.html

Kelesidis, T., & Pothoulakis, C. (2012). Efficacy and safety of the probiotic saccharomyces boulardii for the prevention and therapy of gastrointestinal disorders. *Therapeutic Advances in Gastroenterology*, *5*(2), 111–125. https://doi.org/10.1177/1756283X11428502

Kessler K, Hornemann S, Petzke KJ, Kemper M, Kramer A, Pfeiffer AF, Pivovarova O, Rudovich N. (2017) The effect of diurnal distribution of carbohydrates and fat on glycaemic control in humans: a randomized controlled trial. Sci Rep. 8;7:44170. doi: 10.1038/srep44170.

Knüppel, A., Shipley, M. J., Llewellyn, C. H., & Brunner, E. J. (2017). Sugar intake from sweet food and beverages, common mental disorder and depression: Prospective findings from the whitehall II study. *Scientific Reports*, *7*(1). https://doi.org/10.1038/s41598-017-05649-7

Kochman, J., Jakubczyk, K., Antoniewicz, J., Mruk, H., & Janda, K. (2020). Health benefits and chemical composition of matcha green tea: A review. *Molecules*, *26*(1), 85. https://doi.org/10.3390/molecules26010085

Kota, S., Modi, K., & Satya Krishna, S. (2013). Glycemic variability: Clinical implications. *Indian Journal of Endocrinology and Metabolism*, *17*(4), 611. https://doi.org/10.4103/2230-8210.113751

Kumar, A., Jhilam Pramanik, Goyal, N., Chauhan, D., Nevin Sanlier, Dr. Bhupendra Prajapati, & Chaiyavat Chaiyasut. (2023). Gut microbiota in anxiety and depression: Unveiling the relationships and management options. *Pharmaceuticals*, *16*(4), 565–565. https://doi.org/10.3390/ph16040565

Lazar, S. W., Kerr, C. E., Wasserman, R. H., Gray, J. R., Greve, D. N., Treadway, M. T., McGarvey, M., Quinn, B. T., Dusek, J. A., Benson, H., Rauch, S. L., Moore, C. I., & Fischl, B. (2005). Meditation experience is associated with increased cortical thickness. *Neuroreport*, *16*(17), 1893–1897. https://www.ncbi.nlm.nih.gov/pmc/articles/PMC1361002/

Lee, C.-H., & Giuliani, F. (2019). The role of inflammation in depression and fatigue. *Frontiers in Immunology*, *10*(1696). https://doi.org/10.3389/fimmu.2019.01696

Liemburg-Apers, D. C., Willems, P. H. G. M., Koopman, W. J. H., & Grefte, S. (2015). Interactions between mitochondrial reactive oxygen species and cellular glucose metabolism. *Archives of Toxicology, 89*(8), 1209–1226. https://doi.org/10.1007/s00204-015-1520-y

Liu, P. Z., & Nusslock, R. (2018). Exercise-Mediated neurogenesis in the hippocampus via BDNF. *Frontiers in Neuroscience, 12*(52). https://doi.org/10.3389/fnins.2018.00052

Luo, J. Z., & Luo, L. (2009). Ginseng on hyperglycemia: Effects and mechanisms. *Evidence-Based Complementary and Alternative Medicine, 6*(4), 423–427. https://doi.org/10.1093/ecam/nem178

Ma, X., Nan, F., Liang, H., Shu, P., Fan, X., Song, X., Hou, Y., & Zhang, D. (2022). Excessive intake of sugar: An accomplice of inflammation. *Frontiers in Immunology, 13*(13). https://doi.org/10.3389/fimmu.2022.988481

Manoogian ENC, Chow LS, Taub PR, Laferrère B, Panda S. (2022). Time-restricted Eating for the Prevention and Management of Metabolic Diseases. Endocr Rev. 2022 43(2):405-436. doi: 10.1210/endrev/bnab027.

Maret, W. (2017). Zinc in pancreatic islet biology, insulin sensitivity, and diabetes. *Preventive Nutrition and Food Science, 22*(1), 1–8. https://doi.org/10.3746/pnf.2017.22.1.1

Meng, S., Cao, J., Feng, Q., Peng, J., & Hu, Y. (2013). Roles of chlorogenic acid on regulating glucose and lipids metabolism: A review. *Evidence-Based Complementary and Alternative Medicine, 2013*, 1–11. https://doi.org/10.1155/2013/801457

Mergenthaler, P., Lindauer, U., Dienel, G. A., & Meisel, A. (2013). Sugar for the brain: The role of glucose in physiological and pathological brain function. *Trends in Neurosciences, 36*(10), 587–597. https://doi.org/10.1016/j.tins.2013.07.001

Moreira FD, Reis CEG, Welker AF, Gallassi AD. (2022) Acute Flaxseed Intake Reduces Postprandial Glycemia in Subjects with Type 2 Diabetes: A Randomized Crossover Clinical Trial. Nutrients. 10;14(18):3736. doi: 10.3390/nu14183736.

Mount Sinai. (n.d.). *Omega-6 fatty acids information | Mount Sinai - New York.* Mount Sinai Health System. https://www.mountsinai.org/health-library/supplement/omega-6-fatty-acids

Mroj Alassaf, & Rajan, A. (2023). Diet-induced glial insulin resistance impairs the clearance of neuronal debris in drosophila brain. *PLOS Biology, 21*(11), e3002359–e3002359. https://doi.org/10.1371/journal.pbio.3002359

Mu, Q., Tavella, V. J., & Luo, X. M. (2018). Role of lactobacillus reuteri in human health and diseases. *Frontiers in Microbiology, 9*(757). https://doi.org/10.3389/fmicb.2018.00757

National Institutes of Health. (n.d.). *Office of dietary supplements - dietary supplements for primary mitochondrial disorders.* Ods.od.nih.gov. https://ods.od.nih.gov/factsheets/PrimaryMitochondrialDisorders-HealthProfessional/

National Institutes of Health. (2016). *Office of dietary supplements - magnesium.* National Institutes of Health. https://ods.od.nih.gov/factsheets/Magnesium-HealthProfessional/

National Institutes of Health. (2017). *Office of dietary supplements - dietary supplement fact sheet: Chromium.* Nih.gov.

https://ods.od.nih.gov/factsheets/Chromium-HealthProfessional/

National Institutes of Health. (2021, March 26). *Office of dietary supplements - selenium*. Nih.gov. https://ods.od.nih.gov/factsheets/selenium-healthprofessional/

National Institutes of Health. (2022, October 6). *Office of dietary supplements - calcium.* Nih.gov. https://ods.od.nih.gov/factsheets/Calcium-HealthProfessional/

National Library of Medicine. (1999). Vanadium - help for blood sugar problems? *TreatmentUpdate*, *11*(6), 5–7. https://pubmed.ncbi.nlm.nih.gov/11366936/

Neukirchen, T., Radach, R., & Vorstius, C. (2022). Cognitive glucose sensitivity—proposing a link between cognitive performance and reliance on external glucose uptake. *Nutrition & Diabetes*, *12*(1). https://doi.org/10.1038/s41387-022-00191-6

Norat, P., Soldozy, S., Sokolowski, J. D., Gorick, C. M., Kumar, J. S., Chae, Y., Yağmurlu, K., Prada, F., Walker, M., Levitt, M. R., Price, R. J., Tvrdik, P., & Kalani, M. Y. S. (2020). Mitochondrial dysfunction in neurological disorders: Exploring mitochondrial transplantation. *Npj Regenerative Medicine*, *5*(1). https://doi.org/10.1038/s41536-020-00107-x

Pilcher JJ, Morris DM, Donnelly J, Feigl HB. Interactions between sleep habits and self-control. (2015) Front Hum Neurosci. 11;9:284. doi: 10.3389/fnhum.2015.00284.

Qin, B., Panickar, K. S., & Anderson, R. A. (2010). Cinnamon: Potential role in the prevention of insulin resistance, metabolic syndrome, and type 2 diabetes. *Journal of Diabetes Science and Technology*, 4(3),

685–693.
https://www.ncbi.nlm.nih.gov/pmc/articles/PMC2901047/

Raman, R. (2019, September 26). 6 side effects of too much cinnamon. Healthline; Healthline Media. https://www.healthline.com/nutrition/side-effects-of-cinnamon

Ramezani, M., Fernando, M., Eslick, S., Asih, P. R., Shadfar, S., E.M.S. Bandara, Hillebrandt, H., Silochna Meghwar, Shahriari, M., Chatterjee, P., Thota, R. N., Dias, C. B., Garg, M. L., & Martins, R. N. (2023). Ketone bodies mediate alterations in brain energy metabolism and biomarkers of Alzheimer's disease. *Frontiers in Neuroscience, 17.* https://doi.org/10.3389/fnins.2023.1297984

Robinson MM, Lowe VJ, Nair KS. (2018). Increased Brain Glucose Uptake After 12 Weeks of Aerobic High-Intensity Interval Training in Young and Older Adults. J Clin Endocrinol Metab. 103(1):221-227. doi: 10.1210/jc.2017-01571.

Rodrigues, V. F., Elias-Oliveira, J., Pereira, Í. S., Pereira, J. A., Barbosa, S. C., Machado, M. S. G., & Carlos, D. (2022). Akkermansia muciniphila and gut immune system: A good friendship that attenuates inflammatory bowel disease, obesity, and diabetes. *Frontiers in Immunology, 13.* https://doi.org/10.3389/fimmu.2022.934695

Rodríguez Meléndez, R. (2000). [Importance of biotin metabolism]. *Revista de Investigacion Clinica; Organo Del Hospital de Enfermedades de La Nutricion, 52*(2), 194–199. https://pubmed.ncbi.nlm.nih.gov/10846444/

Rohm, T. V., Meier, D. T., Olefsky, J. M., & Donath, M. Y. (2022). Inflammation in obesity, diabetes, and related disorders.

Immunity, 55(1), 31–55. https://doi.org/10.1016/j.immuni.2021.12.013

Sevinc, G., Rusche, J., Wong, B., Datta, T., Kaufman, R., Gutz, S. E., Schneider, M., Todorova, N., Gaser, C., Thomalla, G., Rentz, D., Dickerson, B. D., & Lazar, S. W. (2021). Mindfulness training improves cognition and strengthens intrinsic connectivity between the hippocampus and posteromedial cortex in healthy older adults. *Frontiers in Aging Neuroscience,* 13. https://doi.org/10.3389/fnagi.2021.702796

Sezer, H., Yazici, D., Copur, S., Dagel, T., Deyneli, O., & Kanbay, M. (2020). The relationship between glycemic variability and blood pressure variability in normoglycemic normotensive individuals. *Blood Pressure Monitoring, Publish Ahead of Print.* https://doi.org/10.1097/mbp.0000000000000491

Sharma, K., Akre, S., Chakole, S., & Wanjari, M. B. (2022). Stress-Induced Diabetes: A Review. *Cureus,* 14(9). https://doi.org/10.7759/cureus.29142

Shishehbor F, Mansoori A, Shirani F. Vinegar consumption can attenuate postprandial glucose and insulin responses; a systematic review and meta-analysis of clinical trials.(2017) Diabetes Res Clin Pract. 127:1-9. doi: 10.1016/j.diabres.2017.01.021.

Shrivastava, S., Sharma, A., Saxena, N., Bhamra, R., & Kumar, S. (2023). Addressing the preventive and therapeutic perspective of berberine against diabetes. *Heliyon,* 9(11), e21233. https://doi.org/10.1016/j.heliyon.2023.e21233

Sleiman, S. F., Henry, J., Al-Haddad, R., El Hayek, L., Abou Haidar, E., Stringer, T., Ulja, D., Karuppagounder, S. S., Holson, E. B., Ratan, R. R., Ninan, I., & Chao, M. V. (2016). Exercise promotes the expression of brain derived neurotrophic factor (BDNF) through the action of the ketone body β-hydroxybutyrate. *ELife*, *5*(e15092). https://doi.org/10.7554/elife.15092

Stull AJ. (2016) Blueberries' Impact on Insulin Resistance and Glucose Intolerance. Antioxidants (Basel). 29;5(4):44. doi: 10.3390/antiox5040044.

Thomas E, Ficarra S, Nakamura M, Drid P, Trivic T, Bianco A. (2024). The Effects of Stretching Exercise on Levels of Blood Glucose: A Systematic Review with Meta-Analysis. Sports Med Open. 10(1):15. doi: 10.1186/s40798-023-00661-w.

Tinsley, G. (2017, May 12). *Top 6 types of creatine reviewed.* Healthline. https://www.healthline.com/nutrition/types-of-creatine

Twarda-Clapa, A., Olczak, A., Białkowska, A. M., & Koziołkiewicz, M. (2022). Advanced glycation end-products (AGEs): Formation, chemistry, classification, receptors, and diseases related to ages. *Cells*, *11*(8), 1312. https://doi.org/10.3390/cells11081312

Uribarri J, Woodruff S, Goodman S, Cai W, Chen X, Pyzik R, Yong A, Striker GE, Vlassara H. (2010). Advanced glycation end products in foods and a practical guide to their reduction in the diet. J Am Diet Assoc. Jun;110(6):911-16.e12. doi: 10.1016/j.jada.2010.03.018.

Vallat R, Shah VD, Walker MP. (2023). Coordinated human sleeping brainwaves map peripheral body glucose homeostasis. Cell Rep Med. 18;4(7):101100. doi: 10.1016/j.xcrm.2023.101100.

Walker, M. P. (2017). Why we sleep: Unlocking the power of sleep and dreams. Scribner, An Imprint Of Simon & Schuster, Inc.

Wani, A. L., Bhat, S. A., & Ara, A. (2015). Omega-3 fatty acids and the treatment of depression: A review of scientific evidence.

Integrative Medicine Research, *4*(3), 132–141. https://doi.org/10.1016/j.imr.2015.07.003

Xiao, X., Luo, Y., & Peng, D. (2022). Updated understanding of the crosstalk between glucose/insulin and cholesterol metabolism. *Frontiers in Cardiovascular Medicine*, *9*. https://doi.org/10.3389/fcvm.2022.879355

Yang, H., Shan, W., Zhu, F., Wu, J., & Wang, Q. (2019). Ketone Bodies in Neurological Diseases: Focus on Neuroprotection and Underlying Mechanisms. *Frontiers in Neurology*, *10*. https://doi.org/10.3389/fneur.2019.00585

Zaplatosch, M. E., & Adams, W. M. (2020). The effect of acute hypohydration on indicators of glycemic regulation, appetite, metabolism and stress: A systematic review and meta-analysis. *Nutrients*, *12*(9), 2526. https://doi.org/10.3390/nu12092526

Zhao, Y., Jia, M., Chen, W., & Liu, Z. (2022). The neuroprotective effects of intermittent fasting on brain aging and neurodegenerative diseases via regulating mitochondrial function. *Free Radical Biology and Medicine*, *182*, 206–218. https://doi.org/10.1016/j.freeradbiomed.2022.02.021

Zeng Y, Wu Y, Zhang Q, Xiao X. (2024). Crosstalk between glucagon-like peptide 1 and gut microbiota in metabolic diseases. mBio. 15(1):e0203223. doi: 10.1128/mbio.02032-23.

Zivkovic, A. M., Telis, N., German, J. B., & Hammock, B. D. (2011). Dietary omega-3 fatty acids aid in the modulation of inflammation and metabolic health. *California Agriculture*, *65*(3), 106–111. https://doi.org/10.3733/ca.v065n03p106

www.ingramcontent.com/pod-product-compliance
Lightning Source LLC
Chambersburg PA
CBHW051729020426
42333CB00014B/1233